CASE REVIEW
Head and Neck Imaging

Series Editor

David M. Yousem, MD
Associate Professor of Radiology, Otorhinolaryngology; Head and Neck Surgery
Department of Radiology
University of Pennsylvania Medical Center
Philadelphia, Pennsylvania

Other Volumes in the CASE REVIEW Series
Brain Imaging
Cardiac Imaging
Gastrointestinal Imaging
General and Vascular Ultrasound
Genitourinary Imaging
Mammography
Musculoskeletal Imaging
Non-vascular Interventional Imaging
Nuclear Medicine
OB/GYN Ultrasound
Pediatric Imaging
Spine Imaging
Thoracic Imaging
Vascular Interventional Imaging

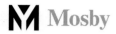

St. Louis Baltimore Boston Carlsbad
Chicago Minneapolis New York Philadelphia Portland
London Milan Sydney Tokyo Toronto

David M. Yousem, MD
Associate Professor of Radiology, Otorhinolaryngology;
   Head and Neck Surgery
Department of Radiology
University of Pennsylvania Medical Center
Philadelphia, Pennsylvania

WITH 348 ILLUSTRATIONS

CASE REVIEW

Head and Neck Imaging

CASE REVIEW SERIES

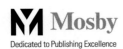

Mosby
Dedicated to Publishing Excellence

A Times Mirror
Company

Publisher: Geoff Greenwood
Editor: Liz Corra
Associate Developmental Editor: Marla Sussman
Project Manager: Linda Clarke
Production Editors: Kathleen Hillock and Jennifer Harper
Designer: Carolyn O'Brien
Manufacturing Manager: William A. Winneberger, Jr.

Copyright © 1998 by Mosby, Inc.

Printed in the United States of America
Composition by Graphic World, Inc.
Printing/binding by Maple-Vail Book Manufacturing Group

Mosby, Inc.
11830 Westline Industrial Drive
St. Louis, Missouri 63146

Library of Congress Cataloging in Publication Data
Yousem, David M.
    Head and neck imaging : case review / David M. Yousem.
      p.   cm.—(Case review series)
    Includes bibliographical references and index.
    ISBN 0-323-00019-3
    1. Head—Imaging—Case studies.   2. Neck—Imaging—Case studies.
I. Title. II. Series.
    [DNLM: 1. Head—radiography examination questions.   2. Neck—
radiography examination questions.   3. Head—radiography case
studies.   4. Neck—radiography case studies.   WE 18.2 Y82h 1998]
RC936.Y68   1998
617.5'1'07572—dc21
DNLM/DLC
for Library of Congress   98-10654
                                     CIP

98 99 00 01 02 / 9 8 7 6 5 4 3 2 1

To the triplets of:
Marilyn, Ilyssa, and Mitch
Mom, Dad, and Sam
Clinical Service, Education, and Research

My experience in teaching medical students, residents, fellows, practicing radiologists, and clinicians has suggested that they love the case conference format more than any other approach. I hope that the reason for this is not a reflection on my lecturing ability, but rather that people stay awake, alert, and on their toes more when they are in the hot seat (or may be the next person to assume the hot seat). In the dozens of continuing medical education courses I have directed, the case review sessions are almost always the most popular parts of the courses.

The idea of this Case Review series grew out of a need for books designed as exam preparation tools for the resident, fellow, or practicing radiologist about to take the boards or the certificate of additional qualification (CAQ) exams. Anxiety runs extremely high concerning the content of these exams, administered as unknown cases. Residents, fellows, and practicing radiologists are very hungry for formats that mimic this exam setting and that cover the types of cases they will encounter and have to accurately describe. In addition, books of this ilk serve as excellent practical reviews of a field and can help a practicing board-certified radiologist keep his or her skills sharpened. Thus heads banged together, and Mosby and I arrived at the format of the volume herein, which is applied consistently to each volume in the series. I hope these volumes strengthen the ability of the reader to interpret studies and apply the knowledge that has been absorbed.

When I started collecting the cases for the first volume of this series on head and neck imaging, researching the entities, and writing the questions and comments, I realized that there were different levels of difficulty that had to be addressed. Therefore I created different sections within the book to acknowledge different degrees of complexity. This organization is applied to all volumes in this Case Review series. There are the Opening Round cases, which graduating radiology residents should have relatively little difficulty mastering. The Fair Game section consists of cases that require more study but most people should get into the ballpark with their differential diagnoses. Finally, there is a Challenge section. I believe that most fellows or fellowship-trained practicing radiologists will be able to mention entities in the differential diagnoses of these challenging cases, but consistently "hitting home runs" will be unlikely. The Challenge cases are really designed to whet one's appetite for further reading on the entities and to test one's wits. Within each of these sections, the selection of cases is entirely random, as one would expect at the boards.

In many instances in these Case Review books, a specific diagnosis may not be what is expected—the quality of the differential diagnosis and the inclusion of appropriate options are most important. Teaching how to distinguish between the diagnostic options (taught in the question and answer and comment sections) will be the goal of the authors of each Case Review volume.

Mosby (through the strong work of Liz Corra) and I have recruited most of the authors of THE REQUISITES™ series (editor, James Thrall, MD) to create Case Review books for their subspecialties. To meet the needs of certain subspecialties and to keep each of the volumes to a consistent, practical size, some specialties will have more than one volume (e.g., ultrasound interventional and vascular radiology, and neuroradiology). Nonetheless, the pleasing tone of THE REQUISITES™ series and its emphasis on condensing the fields of radiology into its foundations will be inculcated into the Case Review volumes. In many situations, THE REQUISITES™ authors have enlisted new coauthors to breathe a novel approach and excitement into the cases submitted. I think the fact that so many of THE REQUISITES™ authors are "on board" for this new series is a testament to their dedication to teaching. I hope that the success of THE REQUISITES™ (series editor, James Thrall, MD) is duplicated with the new Case Review series. Just as THE REQUISITES™ series provides coverage of the essentials in each subspecialty and successfully meets that overwhelming need in the market, I hope that the Case Review series successfully meets the overwhelming need in the market for practical, focused case reviews.

The best way to go through these books is to look at the images, guess the diagnosis, answer the questions, and then turn the page for the answers. If there are two cases on a page, do them two at a time. No peeking!

As for this volume on head and neck imaging, I am afraid that more cases are skewed toward the "challenging" classification simply because most practicing radiologists feel inadequate in assessing lesions in this region. Do not despair! After going through this teaching book, I believe that the reader will find greater confidence and acumen in interpreting studies of head and neck lesions. Perhaps the reader will react as I do when faced with these demanding studies—I wring my hands, scratch my chin, look professional, and give it my best shot . . . with a gleam in my eye. I hope you have fun learning head and neck radiology via the case study approach. I would love your feedback!

David M. Yousem, MD

I have spent my professional career in academic and clinical head and neck imaging. During that time, I have had the opportunity to teach medical students, radiology and otolaryngology residents, neuroradiology fellows, and visiting practicing radiologists. Because I love the teaching experience, I have on numerous occasions thought of the best ways to teach this subject, and I have concluded that several different approaches are necessary to bring the reader from a novice in the field to an accomplished imager. I believe that at one end of the teaching spectrum there is a place for an authoritative text, and to this end Dr. Hugh Curtin and I, in cooperation with Mosby, wrote our two-volume, third edition of *Head and Neck Imaging,* which was published in 1996. This text is intended to be in easy reach on a shelf and used as a reference when specific details on a type of pathology must be referenced or if one wants to try and match the images on a difficult case to images in the book. However, for less experienced radiologists in the field of head and neck imaging, approaching such a formidable text could be a daunting experience that might possibly discourage them from proceeding with their learning of the subspecialty.

To try and reach this audience, a number of smaller books have appeared, each presenting the editor's unique selection of material in a textbook format. Among these more approachable books is the prior effort of Dr. David Yousem and Dr. Robert Grossman in neuroradiology/head and neck imaging, which was published in 1994. This neuroradiology head and neck text, which is part of Mosby's THE REQUISITES™ series (edited by Dr. James Thrall), stands out in my opinion from other similarly sized books because it is both easy to read and full of humor. The authors' theory is that if the learning experience is enjoyable, the reader will endeavor to continue through the entire book and, in the process, learn its contents. This approach has been very favorably judged, as noted by the considerable success of THE REQUISITES™ series. Although that neuroradiology/head and neck text is generally designed as an introduction to the field, the more specific target audience is residents preparing for the radiology boards and radiology fellows and physicians studying for the CAQ examinations.

However, virtually none of these previous textbooks is presented in a format that recreates how radiology is actually practiced—namely, reading a series of individual cases. Such a case-oriented approach simulates not only everyday clinical radiology, but also the way cases are presented at examinations such as the boards and the CAQs. In this new book, Dr. Yousem has combined such a case-oriented approach with the humor he introduced in *Neuroradiology: THE REQUISITES.* His desire is to provide the reader with a selection of cases of graduated difficulty that will prepare one for accurate interpretation of head and neck imaging studies in the office and at the boards. The key to holding the reader's attention is a well-edited choice of cases presented with succinct, incisive commentary that is used to stimulate one to forge on through the entire text. Key questions on each case are asked, and the answers are presented with recent references. As a further learning experience, this new book is cross-referenced to *Neuroradiology: THE REQUISITES* so that the reader can easily pursue further details on particular questions.

Dr. Yousem, whom I have known for about 8 years, is one of a group of young, bright radiologists who, to my delight, are very devoted to academics and teaching. David also has a unique and enjoyable sense of humor that he brings to these books, and I believe that his new book, designed to be part of the new Case Review series (edited by Dr. David Yousem), will be a successful text that teaches, prepares one for examinations in head and neck imaging, and lightens the task of studying.

I earnestly hope that David's book stimulates more people to learn and take up the challenge of the field of head and neck imaging. In addition, I salute his efforts and his wife Marilyn's tolerance. I am sure that the reader will both learn from and enjoy this book.

Peter M. Som, MD, FACR

This book was born out of a love and a need.

A love. I love interpreting studies of the head and neck because of its complexity and nuances. A need. We need a head and neck radiology Case Review book along the lines of Doug Yock's *Magnetic Resonance Imaging of the Central Nervous System Disease: A Teaching File* (Mosby) to prepare for the neuroradiology CAQ. I enjoyed his book and learned so much from it. Until someone writes the definitive "Yockesque" head and neck case book, this book may suffice.

It was not until a neuroradiologist from Porto, Portugal, Alexandra Campos-Lopes, visited me for 2 weeks in December 1996 that I realized I was *able* to write this book. Over her 2-week visit, we spent hours poring over head and neck cases together as I tried to provide a crash course on head and neck radiology. By the end of this time, we had literally gone over hundreds of cases, good quality cases, and I thought to myself, "I *can* do it. And I *want* to do it. Now how can I convince Marilyn (my wife) to *let me* do it?"

"Now how can I convince Marilyn to *let me* do it?" What an exaggeration. Never has there been a more supportive wife than Marilyn. She has endured (very recently, actually) weeks of having her husband out of the country lecturing or "conferencing" or, even worse, physically remote while in the same house as he pored over his computer, oblivious to all, trying to find the right question to stimulate the reader. I never had to convince Marilyn to let me write this book—she was all for it, and I think she enjoys seeing me show as much enthusiasm for my work as I do for the other important parts of my life, fatherdom and husbandhood.

In writing this book I learned how complete and incomplete *Neuroradiology: THE REQUISITES,* coauthored by Bob Grossman and myself, is. There are entities in this Case Review book that do not appear in our larger text, so some references to THE REQUISITES™ volume get you into the anatomic area but do not explicitly discuss the lesion. Hopefully, by directing you to the right pages in our REQUISITES™ textbook, you will be able to learn why a lesion is *not* some of the other entities in the region, and you will be able to broaden or narrow some of your differential diagnoses. This Case Review book has also inspired me in the writing of the second edition of *Neuroradiology: THE REQUISITES* (and my enthusiasm has inspired Bob Grossman as well, so we are back in the studio "cutting our next edition"!). In a similar vein, most of the articles from the literature that I cite are not the "classics" in the field. I have tried to emphasize the most recent literature with the expectation that the most recent papers might shed new light on an entity and have in their bibliographies some of the more classic descriptions of the lesions.

I want to thank all of the residents and fellows who through the years have given me a sense of what makes a good case and what questions are appropriate to ask what level of trainee. Their boundless enthusiasm is always inspiring. I want to thank Alexandra Campos-Lopes and the radiology residents rotating through neuroradiology in November and December 1996, Maj Wickstrom and Bamidele Kammen, for helping to motivate me to write this book. Thanks also go to Adam Flanders and Joel Swartz, who reviewed the case material and provided pointed suggestions for improving the manuscript. I want to thank Laurie Loevner, my partner (and close friend) in head and neck radiology and neuroradiology at the University of Pennsylvania Medical Center. Without Laurie taking some of the work load off my shoulders and providing some of the outstanding cases in the book, I probably could not have pulled this off as quickly and (hopefully) as effectively as I have. Plus, her insights into each case demonstrate her eminence in the field of head and neck radiology.

I want to thank Liz Corra, who negotiated with me to write a book and edit a series that fulfilled my needs, Mosby's needs, and the market's needs. Liz has become a very good friend and my best e-mail pen pal. She has been an enthusiastic supporter of this project, and the series it has inspired, the Case Review series. I needed very little encouragement throughout the writing of this book because in general it was much more enjoyable than writing a "dry" textbook (even with the amount of humor we tried to incorporate into *Neuroradiology: THE REQUISITES*), but Liz provided it.

To Bob Grossman, my friend, confidant, and coauthor, I express my appreciation for giving me the opportunity to write this book, at least partly on company time. Bob and I have gotten out all the joke books and Ogden Nash collections for the second edition of *Neuroradiology: THE REQUISITES.*

To friends and colleagues on the clinical side—David Kennedy, Randy Weber, Ara Chalian, Andy Goldberg, Erica Thaler, Greg Weinstein, Doug Bigelow, Glen Knox, Don Lanza, Mark Kotapka, Gene Flamm, Eric Zager, Kevin Judy—and on the neuroradiology/head and neck radiology side—Bob Grossman, David Hackney, Linda Bagley, Bob Hurst, Laurie Loevner, Joe Maldjian, Herb Goldberg, Frank Lexa, Hugh Curtin, Peter Som, Patty Hudgins, among many—thanks for the help.

I would also like to give credit to *Head and Neck Imaging,* third edition, edited by Peter Som and Hugh Curtin and published by Mosby. This is the ultimate head and neck imaging reference book, and I found myself gravitating to that book for the discussion and questions on many of the entities herein. I do not cite the book as a "reference" per se, but I believe every radiologist who interprets head and neck studies should have this book within arm's reach.

It seems just yesterday that I was dedicating a book to my "daughter Ilyssa and in utero son." If you could see Ilyssa now, curly, beautiful, and in her gymnastics prime at age 6. And Mitchell, 3½ and all boy with Buzz Lightyear (he calls it "Buzz Lightning") dolls, trucks galore, and a particular knack for puzzles (a reconstructive surgeon in the making?). Thanks to my cherished wife to whom I come home and who keeps me whole: "You complete me." And to my supportive family and friends to whom I do not come home, but who I always know are out there: Nana, Zaydie, Tess, Sam, Penny, Laurie, John, Peter, Beth, Barry, Mel, Scott, and so on.

I hope you like the book.

David M. Yousem, MD

Opening Round

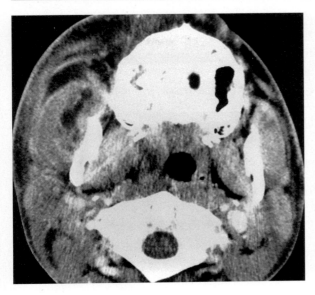 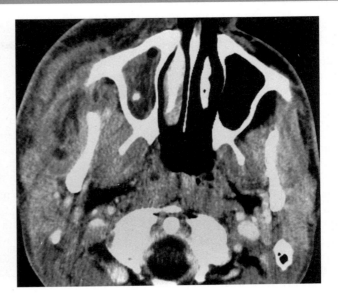

1. In what space is the lesion?

2. What are the common sources of inflammatory lesions in this space?

3. What are the findings that suggest this lesion is inflammatory as opposed to neoplastic?

4. What cranial nerve serves as a conduit from the masticator space to the intracranial compartment?

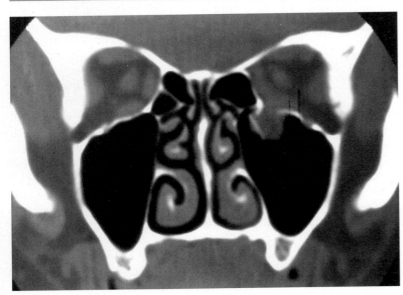

1. Which is more likely to fracture, the orbital floor or the rim? Why?

2. What may herniate through the gap of a floor fracture?

3. Looking which way increases the diplopia with entrapped muscles or fat associated with a floor fracture?

4. How often do orbital floor and medial wall fractures coexist?

CASE 1

Masticator Space Abscess

1. The masticator space.

2. Odontogenic (dental) infections, iatrogenic (surgical) manipulation, sialadenitis or sialolithiasis of the submandibular gland, and tonsillitis.

3. Infiltration of the subcutaneous fat, thickening of the skin, and absence of central/solid contrast enhancement.

4. The trigeminal (fifth) cranial nerve (mandibular V-3 division).

Reference

Hardin CW, Harnsberger HR, Osborn AG, Doxey GP, Davis RK, Nyberg DA: Infection and tumor of the masticator space: CT evaluation, *Radiology* 157:413-417, 1985.

Cross-Reference

Neuroradiology: THE REQUISITES, pp 424-429.

Comment

One knows that this lesion is in the masticator space because the prestyloid parapharyngeal fat is displaced medially and posteriorly. The enlargement of the right masseter and pterygoid muscles on either side of the mandible also clearly identifies the location of the lesion, and the low density area within the right masseter muscle suggests an abscess. The main roles of CT with regard to masticator space inflammatory lesions are to define whether an abscess exists (suitable for drainage) and to search for evidence of osteomyelitis. Abscesses are defined collections usually seen with rim or ring enhancement. Cellulitis, myositis, and fasciitis do not have discrete collections to drain. From the masticator space, infections can spread to the base of the skull, the temporomandibular joint, the floor of the mouth, or the upper neck. The importance of identifying osteomyelitis of the mandible or maxilla lies in the prolonged antibiotic therapy required to eradicate the infection in the bone. With respect to diagnosing osteomyelitis of the mandible, I think that nuclear scintigraphy and MRI do a better job than CT. Dental amalgam is the bane of CT (and less so MRI)—it can totally obscure odontogenic lesions and mandibular erosions in adjacent bone. Angled CT scanning in multiple planes can sometimes help—other times you just have to wring your hands and give it your best shot.

Bottom line: Brush your teeth and see a dentist twice a year. (Sponsored by the ADA.)

Notes

CASE 2

Left Orbital Floor Fracture (Old)

1. The floor fractures first because it is composed of slightly thinner bone and the pressure is transmitted to the inside of the orbit where the floor is.

2. Fat, the inferior rectus muscle, the inferior oblique muscle, or the medial rectus muscle—in that order.

3. Upward gaze.

4. Fifty percent of the time, though they may be subtle and only at the inferomedial margin of the orbit.

Reference

Sullivan WG: Displaced orbital roof fractures: presentation and treatment, *Plast Reconstr Surg* 87:657-661, 1991.

Cross-Reference

Neuroradiology: THE REQUISITES, pp 165-167.

Comment

The sine qua non of orbital floor fractures is the air-fluid level in the ipsilateral maxillary antrum. Absence of this finding might suggest the injury is old or that the herniated orbital contents have tamponaded the bleeding site. Surprisingly, there is often very little orbital emphysema with floor fractures; this may be due to the sealant effect of the herniated material into the defect that communicates with the maxillary antrum. Plastic, trauma, or ear, nose, and throat surgeons tend to fight over these types of cases; all agree, however, that when imaging studies show entrapment or enophthalmos, the patient's orbit should probably be repaired. The floor can be repaired with native bone or alloplasts—often meshlike material that supports the orbital contents and is nonresorbable.

A rise in intraorbital pressure leads to the floor fracture. Why is the orbital floor more susceptible to fractures than the orbital roof? After all, they have similar thicknesses. The predilection for the floor to fracture arises from its natural weakness, which is caused by the presence of the infraorbital nerve and canal in the floor. The arched shape of the roof spares it from the full effect of the increased intraorbital pressure.

The terms *trap door* and *bomb-bay door* are sometimes used to refer to the configuration of the fracture fragments as they prolapse into the superior maxillary antrum.

Notes

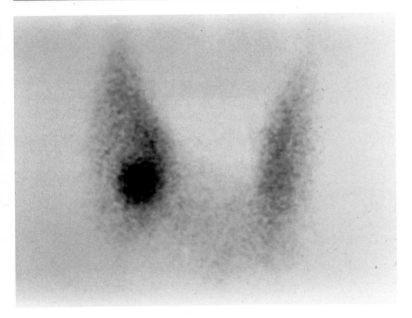

1. What is Plummer's disease?
2. How does one distinguish an autonomous nodule from one that is "hypertrophic"?
3. At what size do autonomous nodules begin to cause hyperthyroidism?
4. Besides autonomous and hypertrophic functioning "hot" nodules, what else can be hot?

CASE 4

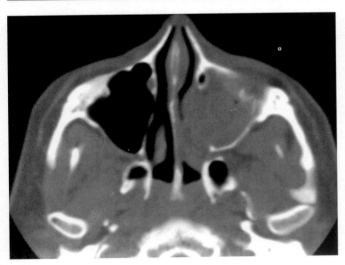 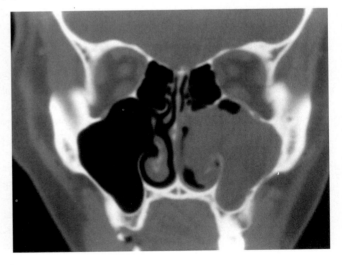

1. Provide a differential diagnosis for a unilateral polypoid mass in the paranasal sinus.
2. Bilateral polypoid masses in the sinuses would include what diagnoses?
3. What are the MRI characteristics of antrochoanal polyps?
4. What are the demographics of antrochoanal polyps?

Hot Nodule on Thyroid Scintigraphy

1. Hyperthyroidism caused by a solitary autonomous hot nodule.

2. The difference between the two depends on the lesion's response to a thyroid suppression test. If the lesion suppresses, it is functional (hypertrophic) and under hormonal feedback control. If it continues to secrete even after thyroid hormone administration, it is autonomous.

3. They usually have to be over 3 cm in size to cause symptoms.

4. Areas of thyroiditis, diffuse toxic goiter (Graves' disease), multinodular toxic goiter, and (very, very rarely) a thyroid cancer.

Reference

Yousem DM, Scheff A: Thyroid and parathyroid gland pathology: role of imaging, *Otolaryngol Clin North Am* 28:621-650, 1995.

Cross-Reference

Neuroradiology: THE REQUISITES, p 440.

Comment

Hyperthyroidism is most commonly caused by Graves' disease (diffuse toxic goiter), multinodular toxic goiters, and hot solitary nodules. Struma ovarii (ectopic thyroid tissue in the ovary) and thyroiditis are rarer causes of hyperthyroidism. Suppression with administration of exogenous thyroid hormone is the treatment used if the toxic adenoma is merely hypertrophic and not autonomous. If it is autonomous and is causing hyperthyroidism, the option of iodine ablation or surgical removal can be discussed. A zebra entity is Marine-Lenhart disease—Graves' disease with hyperplastic nonautonomous nodules. In this case the "Graves'" pattern is modified to show not only increased uptake and an enlarged gland, but also cold nodules within that gland (from suppressed hypertrophic nodules caused by the Graves' outpouring of thyroid hormones).

An autonomous nodule over 4 cm in size usually causes suppression of the remainder of the thyroid gland through the pituitary gland's feedback control with thyroid stimulating hormone (TSH). If the nodule is 1 to 2 cm in size, one may see normal thyroid gland radiotracer uptake in the background of the hot nodule. Less than 1% of hot nodules harbor cancers.

(Bet you never thought there would be radioactive nukes in this book. Surprise!)

Notes

Antrochoanal Polyp

1. Inverted papilloma, antrochoanal polyp, allergic polyposis, allergic fungal sinusitis, juvenile angiofibroma, fungus ball (mycetoma), mucoceles, granuloma, and mucous retention cyst.

2. Allergic or inflammatory polyposis, cystic fibrosis, fungus balls.

3. Bright on T2W scans, peripheral gadolinium enhancement, well-defined masses located in the maxillary antrum extending into the nasal choana, expansion of these cavities.

4. Young male adults (most <40 years old), sometimes with a history of allergies.

Reference

Cook PR, Davis WE, McDonald R, McKinsey JP: Antrochoanal polyposis: a review of 33 cases, *Ear Nose Throat J* 72: 401-411, 1993.

Cross-Reference

Neuroradiology: THE REQUISITES, p 369.

Comment

Most cases of antrochoanal polyps that I have seen have been solitary unilateral masses that have not occurred within a background of sinonasal polyposis. These appear to be isolated masses, and when they are solitary I suggest this diagnosis over the myriad of polyps that can occur in the sinonasal cavity. The cause may still be obstruction of the ostiomeatal complex, as opposed to a response to allergens. Others disagree, noting the 10% incidence of antrochoanal polyps in a setting of allergic polyposis. The lesions arise from the lining of the maxillary sinus and comprise 3% to 6% of all sinonasal polyps. Recurrence rates are as high as 25%. No malignant potential is present.

Papillomas in the nose are usually separated into 3 types: inverted papillomas, fungiform papillomas, and cylindric cell papillomas. Most papillomas are fungiform, which are associated (as are inverted papillomas) with human papillomaviruses. Fungiform papillomas usually arise from the nasal septum and are unilateral and solitary, whereas inverted papillomas usually arise from the lateral nasal wall. Cylindric cell papillomas are the least common type of papillomas, and they also arise from the lateral nasal wall. Only inverted papillomas are associated with concomitant malignancies.

Notes

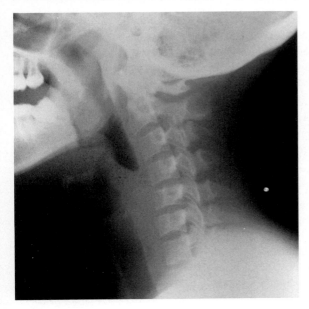

1. What is the stereotypical organism associated with this diagnosis?
2. How do adult and pediatric versions of this infection differ?
3. Why do some people use the term *supraglottitis* rather than *epiglottitis?*
4. Why do people not use CT to diagnose this entity?

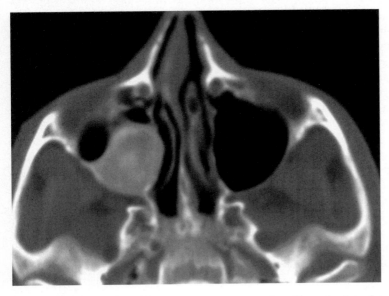

1. What are the facial bones most commonly affected with this entity?
2. Define Albright's syndrome.
3. What is the term used for gross polyostotic diffuse fibrous dysplasia involvement of the facial bones?
4. How frequently is there malignant degeneration of fibrous dysplasia?

Epiglottitis

1. *Haemophilus influenzae* type B.

2. *Streptococcus* may predominate as the organism in adults. The infection is milder in adults and is less likely to cause acute respiratory arrest or obstruction. (This may be due to the larger airway diameter in adults.)

3. The aryepiglottic folds and arytenoids may be primarily involved, not just the epiglottis. In some cases the soft palate and prevertebral swelling may be the predominant factors in creating upper respiratory symptoms.

4. The risk of airway compromise is too great when scanning a patient in the supine position. Usually, only plain films with the patient in the erect position are taken (if any imaging at all is required).

Reference

Nemzek WR, Katzberg RW, Van Slyke MA, Bickley LS: A reappraisal of the radiologic findings of acute inflammation of the epiglottis and supraglottic structures in adults, *AJNR Am J Neuroradiol* 16:495-502, 1995.

Cross-Reference

Neuroradiology: THE REQUISITES, pp 387, 395.

Comment

Adult supraglottitis is making a comeback, possibly because of the acquired immunodeficiency syndrome (AIDS) epidemic. It has returned as a more indolent infection than pediatric epiglottitis because adults can tolerate more supraglottic and prevertebral swelling than children. The width of the epiglottis in an adult should be less than one third of the anteroposterior width of the C4 vertebral body. Likewise, the width of the prevertebral tissues in an adult should be less than one half of the anteroposterior width of the C4 vertebral body. Epiglottitis occurs most commonly in the winter and has a bimodal age distribution of 0 to 8 years old and 20 to 40 years old. Fever, drooling, sore throat pain, dysphagia, stridor, and tachypnea are common. Two classic findings on lateral plain films are (1) the epiglottis that looks like a thumbprint because of its thickness and (2) hypopharyngeal distention caused by airway obstruction. Anteroposterior plain films are only performed if croup is in the differential diagnosis. Croup occurs in young children (<2 years old) and is usually a viral illness. Pain is not a typical finding, and dysphagia is unusual with croup. The "steeple" sign of laryngeal narrowing can be seen on anteroposterior plain film views of the airway of a patient with croup.

Notes

Fibrous Dysplasia of the Maxilla

1. The maxilla (more so than the mandible), the zygoma, and the bones of the sinonasal cavity. The sphenoid bone (greater wing more so than lesser wing) and the base of the skull may also be involved.

2. Precocious puberty and polyostotic fibrous dysplasia usually found in young girls. The patients have café au lait spots that resemble the coast of Maine in that they have irregular borders.

3. Leontiasis ossea.

4. Less than 1%; however, the rate is increased with involvement of the skull and facial bones and with *polyostotic* fibrous dysplasia.

Reference

Jee WH, Choi KH, Choe BY, Park JM, Shinn KS: Fibrous dysplasia: MR imaging characteristics with radiopathologic correlation, *AJR Am J Roentgenol* 167:1523-1527, 1996.

Cross-Reference

Neuroradiology: THE REQUISITES, pp 390, 425.

Comment

The T2W signal intensity characteristics of fibrous dysplasia are variable, with one third to one half dark and one half to two thirds bright. One may find septations, cysts, hemorrhagic products, and extraosseous extension. Enhancement may be homogeneous (three fourths) or rimlike (one fourth). The differential diagnosis includes ossifying fibromas, fibroxanthoma (dark on T1W and T2W scans), malignant fibrous histiocytoma, and Paget's disease. A ground glass appearance on plain films or CT is most characteristic of fibrous dysplasia, and the absence of cortical thickening is more typical of fibrous dysplasia than the other leading differential diagnosis, Paget's disease. Of course, one typically does not consider Paget's disease until the patient is into the sixth decade of life, and fibrous dysplasia is a disease affecting young adults. An association with myxomas has been reported with fibrous dysplasia.

Fibrous dysplasia can be lytic (21%), sclerotic (homogeneously dense) (23%), and pagetoid (ground glass) (56%) and may involve the skull in virtually any location.

Rarely one may see manifestations of metastatic disease or osseous changes associated with meningiomas that may simulate fibrous dysplasia of the sphenoid bones. In the maxilla, as in this case, one should at the very least be sure that the lesion is not somehow of odontogenic origin because some dental lesions (e.g., cherubism, adenomatoid lesions) may also look like fibrous dysplasia.

Notes

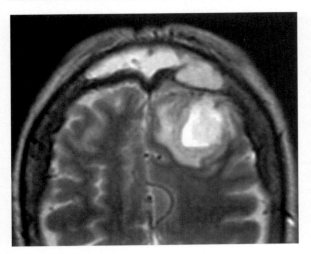 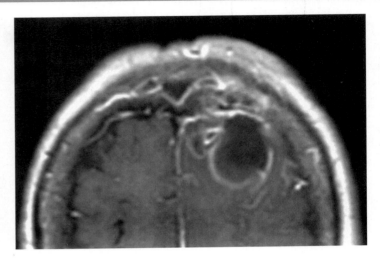

1. What MRI characteristics suggest that this lesion is inflammatory rather than neoplastic?

2. What sinonasal neoplasm is associated with intracranial cysts that might appear similar to those on this patient's study?

3. How are frontal sinuses obliterated?

4. How often does one experience intracranial complications of sinusitis?

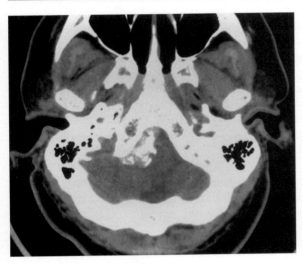 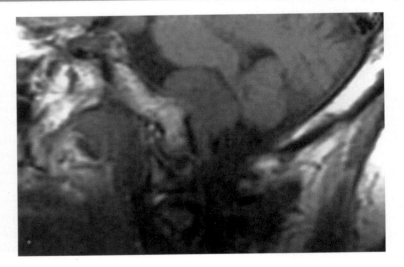

1. What does the differential diagnosis of a calcified skull base mass include?

2. Without the calcification, what else should be considered in the differential diagnosis of this lesion?

3. Is there an increase in the frequency of meningiomas in patients with neurofibromatosis?

4. What is the most common radiation-induced CNS neoplasm? Does it have any unique characteristics?

Frontal Sinusitis with Meningitis and Abscess

1. The rim enhancement and hyperintensity on T2W scans.

2. Olfactory neuroblastoma.

3. The frontoethmoidal recess is plugged with fascia, methyl methacrylate, bone, or muscle. The sinus is usually stuffed with fat. The mucosa of the sinus is stripped.

4. Unless one considers headaches to be an intracranial complication, less than 1% of all patients with sinusitis develop central nervous system (CNS) problems.

Reference

Loevner LA, Yousem DM, Lanza DC, Kennedy DW, Goldberg AN: MR evaluation of frontal sinus osteoplastic flaps with autogenous fat grafts, *AJNR Am J Neuroradiol* 16:1721-1726, 1995.

Cross-Reference

Neuroradiology: THE REQUISITES, pp 174-176, 299-300, 368-369.

Comment

In up to 40% of asymptomatic individuals (depending on the season and where they live), there are changes compatible with acute or chronic sinusitis evident on CT or MRI. By the same token, about 15% to 20% of patients with sinus symptoms have negative imaging studies. At endoscopy about 10% of patients determined to be "totally normal" by imaging studies have significant sinus mucosal findings. Most cases of sinusitis do not necessitate imaging of any kind except through the endoscope. Imaging is used predominantly to guide surgery or to assess for intraorbital or intracranial extension of the infection. Intraorbital infection is probably evaluated equally well with either CT or MRI, but certainly MRI is the gold standard for evaluating intracranial and optic nerve pathology related to sinusitis.

Besides meningitis (seen here as dural enhancement) and abscess formation (periosteal, epidural, or subdural empyemas), one should consider venous and dural sinus thrombosis and thrombophlebitis as possible causes of neurologic complications of sinusitis. Arteritis and mycotic aneurysm formation are not commonly seen except in cases of the most virulent fungal infections.

Notes

Meningioma at Skull Base

1. Meningioma, chordoma, chondrosarcoma, granulomatous disease, and aneurysm.

2. Dural metastases, sarcoidosis, granulomatous infections (tuberculous, fungal, Langerhans' cell histiocytosis), lymphoma, schwannoma, and dural plasmacytomas.

3. Yes, particularly with neurofibromatosis type 2.

4. A meningioma. The radiation-induced meningiomas are more aggressive, recur more frequently, grow faster, undergo malignant degeneration more commonly, and have more mitoses and a higher metabolic rate than de novo meningiomas.

Reference

Tsuchiya K, Hachiya J, Mizutani Y, Yoshino A: Three-dimensional helical CT angiography of skull base meningiomas, *AJNR Am J Neuroradiol* 17:933-936, 1996.

Cross-Reference

Neuroradiology: THE REQUISITES, pp 68-73, 509-510.

Comment

The skull base is one of the locations where one can justify scanning lesions with both CT and MRI. Surgeons need the soft tissue resolution of MRI to see the relationship between lesions and the cranial nerves, the brain, and the nearby vascular structures. CT is most useful for viewing bony landmarks and anatomic variants that guide or hinder surgery. In addition, angiography with embolization or interventional management of the arterial and venous structures may be necessary. MR angiography and CT arteriography have successfully made inroads into the diagnostic imaging of the relationship between masses and the vascular structures. Three-dimensional imaging may even guide surgery with intraoperative localization. Relationships may be more easily displayed with three-dimensional data sets.

Meningiomas come in many different varieties, including the fibroblastic, transitional, syncytial, angioblastic, and malignant anaplastic types—with aggressiveness increasing in that order. On T2W scans the syncytial and angioimmunoblastic types are often brighter than the fibroblastic and transitional types. Meningiomas are the most common type of nonglial brain tumor and are usually well managed surgically. Recurrent or primary skull base meningiomas that have failed conventional surgical therapy may be treated successfully with radiation therapy with or without brachytherapy with interstitial iodine-125 seeds.

Notes

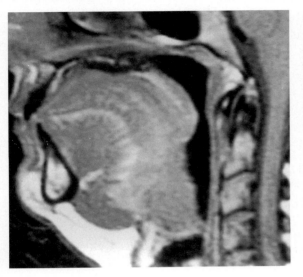
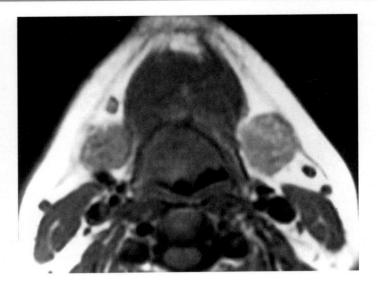

1. Where is this lesion located?
2. What factors are associated with nonneoplastic lymphoid enlargement of Waldeyer's ring?
3. How can this lesion be distinguished from lymphoma?
4. What findings on a sagittal scout T1W MRI suggest human immunodeficiency virus (HIV) positivity?

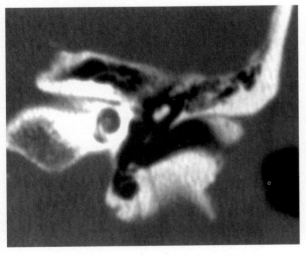
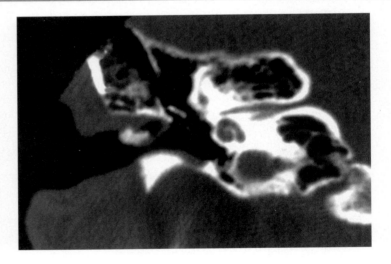

1. Describe the typical patient who has these lesions.
2. To what lesions are patients with external auditory exostoses more susceptible?
3. Distinguish external auditory canal cholesteatomas from keratosis obturans.
4. With what is keratosis obturans associated?

CASE 9

Lymphoid Hyperplasia of the Lingual Tonsil

1. The base of the tongue, specifically within the lingual tonsil.

2. Chronic inflammation and irritation (Beware you smokers!), HIV positivity, mononucleosis (chronic Epstein-Barr virus [EBV] infection), and youth (<20 to 30 years old).

3. Lymphoid hyperplasia and lymphoma of the tongue base often look exactly alike. If there are infiltrative margins beyond the expected location of the circumvallate papillae, or there is deep tongue invasion, one should suggest lymphoma. Lymphadenopathy may or may not be helpful because young individuals often have hyperplastic nodes.

4. The constellation of (1) nasopharyngeal adenoidal tissue prominence, (2) abnormal bone marrow signal, (3) posterior triangle lymphadenopathy, and (4) intraparotid cysts and/or nodes strongly suggests HIV positivity.

Reference

Yousem DM, Loevner LA, Tobey JD, Bilker WB, Chalian AA: Adenoidal width and HIV factors, *AJNR Am J Neuroradiol* 18:1721-1725, 1997.

Cross-Reference

Neuroradiology: THE REQUISITES, pp 384-385.

Comment

Lymphoid hypertrophy may be a normal response to chronic irritants in the oral/oropharyngeal cavity. However, it may cause symptoms such as those associated with sleep apnea. Recommending a biopsy to exclude a lymphoma for someone who ends up having lymphoid hyperplasia is one of the expected hazards of head and neck radiology.

The cause of lymphoid hypertrophy in HIV-positive patients is somewhat controversial. No direct correlation between lymphoid thickness and white blood cell counts or CD4 counts has been shown. Histopathologically, one finds follicular hyperplasia with large and irregular germinal centers, thinning of the mantle zones, HIV virus particles, HIV antigens, and markers for viral RNA within germinal centers or on the mucosal surface. The findings in Waldeyer's ring are often associated with hyperplastic lymph nodes that also have follicular hyperplasia within them. The lymphoid tissue in the nodes and adenoids may serve as a filter for the virus and associated immune complexes, but inadvertently it may also be a route for greater dissemination of the HIV virus if retained viral particles (and RNA) pass into the lymphocytes. The findings of lymphoid hyperplasia are most commonly seen in the adenoids, nodes, palatine tonsils, and lingual tonsils (in descending order).

Notes

CASE 10

Bilateral External Auditory Canal Exostoses

1. Cold water swimmers.

2. Keratosis obturans and cholesteatomas.

3. Keratosis obturans is usually bilateral, seen in younger individuals, and more painful than external auditory canal cholesteatomas.

4. Bronchiectasis, obstructive plugs in the external auditory canals, sinusitis.

Reference

Fisher EW, McManus TC: Surgery for external auditory canal exostoses and osteomata, *J Laryngol Otol* 108:106-110, 1994.

Cross-Reference

Neuroradiology: THE REQUISITES, pp 336-338.

Comment

Cold water swimmers really do get external auditory canal exostoses. The length of exposure is usually years of this type of swimming. The Scandinavian, New Zealand, and Australian literature is replete with studies of these crazy arctic/antarctic skinny-dippers who develop the exostoses. Even after surgical removal of the exostoses (and psychological counseling), patients who return to their "polar bear club" cold water habits develop new exostoses. (Personally, I'm more the hot tub kind of guy!) Patients may also develop external otitis that brings them in to their doctors, or they may have meatal blockage. The differential diagnosis includes keratosis obturans, epidermoids, acquired cholesteatomas, polyps, and osteomas. Osteomas are usually pedunculated and more lateral than exostoses, and they contain stroma. True exostoses are sessile, flat, and medial, and contain dense lamellar bone without fibrovascular spaces. The other lesions (keratosis obturans, epidermoids, polyps, and cholesteatomas) do not usually calcify/ossify.

Notes

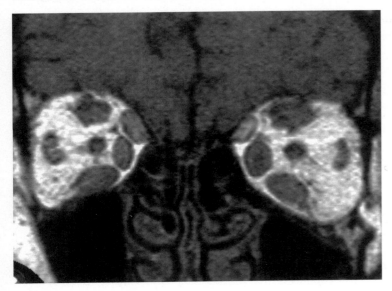

1. What is the major indication for decompression in a patient who has this disease?

2. What rectus muscle is least likely to be affected by thyroid ophthalmopathy?

3. In a patient who has AIDS and a dense globe, what is the differential diagnosis?

4. In what percentage of patients with sarcoidosis are there orbital findings? What are the most common manifestations of orbital sarcoidosis?

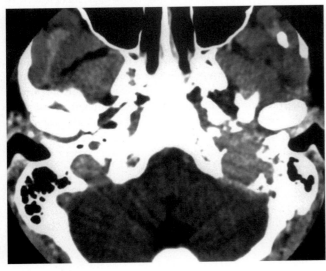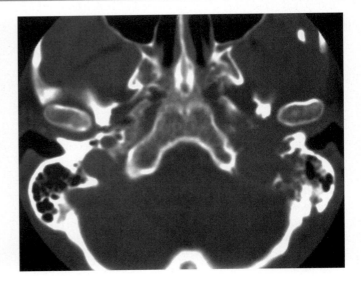

1. What are Arnold's and Jacobson's nerves?

2. Does a glomus jugulare usually arise from the pars nervosa or pars vascularis of the jugular foramen?

3. How often is the jugular vein involved with a glomus jugulare?

4. What is the nuclear medicine agent that currently is most accurate for detecting multiple paragangliomas?

Thyroid Eye Disease

1. Optic nerve compression and/or ischemia secondary to enlarged extraocular muscles.

2. The lateral rectus muscle.

3. Hemorrhagic retinitis, cytomegalovirus retinitis, retinal detachments, and silicone oil retinopexy (for treatment of retinitis).

4. Forty-five percent. Involved structures may include the ciliary body, choroid, and/or iris (uveitis), retina, conjunctiva, lacrimal gland, optic nerve, extraocular muscles, optic chiasm, meninges, or the optic pathways.

Reference

Birchall D, Goodall KL, Noble JL, Jackson A: Graves' ophthalmopathy: intracranial fat prolapse on CT images as an indicator of optic nerve compression, *Radiology* 200:123-127, 1996.

Cross-Reference

Neuroradiology: THE REQUISITES, p 296.

Comment

One must remember that the patient need not be hyperthyroid to have Graves' ophthalmopathy (thyroid eye disease). This is the most common cause of unilateral or bilateral proptosis in adults, presumably because of increased orbital fat and extraocular muscle enlargement. Classically the tendinous insertions are spared in thyroid eye disease but affected with idiopathic orbital pseudotumor. Optic neuropathy occurs in 5% of patients with thyroid eye disease as a result of compression and ischemic insult at the orbital apex. Visual loss can occur precipitously, so patients are screened carefully for optic pathology. Intracranial fat prolapse across the plane of the superior orbital fissure and optic nerve crowding with greater than 50% effacement of perineural fat are the best predictors of Graves'-related optic neuropathy. In a patient with unilateral single muscle enlargement, one should include myositis caused by adjacent inflammatory sinusitis, pseudotumor, thyroid eye disease, myxoma, rhabdomyo(sarco)ma, schwannoma, intramuscular hematoma, sarcoidosis, lymphoma, and metastases in the differential diagnosis.

Approximately 7% of patients with Graves' disease manifest proptosis and protrusion of ocular fat without muscular enlargement. The relationship between clinical findings of diplopia or ophthalmoplegia and the presence of muscular enlargement is actually fairly weak, particularly with early Graves' disease. Rarely, one may also see fatty infiltration of the muscle, suggested in the superior oblique of this patient's left orbit.

Notes

Glomus Jugulare

1. Arnold's nerve is the auricular branch of the vagus nerve, and Jacobson's nerve is the jugulotympanic branch of the glossopharyngeal nerve.

2. Pars vascularis.

3. Almost 100% of the time.

4. Indium-111 octreotide.

Reference

Watkins LD, Mendoza N, Cheesman AD, Symon L: Glomus jugulare tumors: a review of 61 cases, *Acta Neurochir* 130:66-70, 1994.

Cross-Reference

Neuroradiology: THE REQUISITES, p 332.

Comment

Deafness and/or tinnitus usually cause the patient with a glomus tumor to seek professional help, and the neurootologist usually picks up cranial nerve palsies on exam. The otologists (middle ear lesions) and neurosurgeons (skull base infiltrative lesion) fight over who gets to resect these cases, and usually there is a little something for the neurointerventional radiologist as well (for preoperative embolization or to detect those subtle subcentimeter additional paragangliomas). Radiation therapy often stops progression of a glomus jugulare but does not make it regress. Catecholamine secretion occurs in only about 4% of cases, and urinary vanillylmandelic acid and metanephrines should be collected. Neural infiltration by glomus jugulare tumors affects the vagus nerve in 61% of cases; the facial, glossopharyngeal, and spinal accessory nerves in 50%; and the hypoglossal nerve in 36%. The differential diagnosis of a hypervascular erosive jugular foramen mass includes hemangiopericytomas, metastases (kidney and thyroid), meningiomas, granular cell tumors, angiofibromas, endolymphatic sac tumors, and plasmacytomas. Schwannomas and nasopharyngeal masses growing into the jugular foramen, although more common than some of the zebras listed above, are not hypervascular at angiography.

Notes

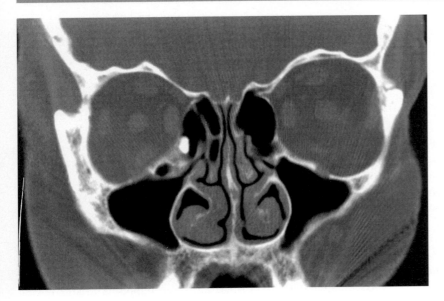

1. What is a Haller cell?

2. What is the significance of a Haller cell?

3. What is the incidence of osteoma in all patients who present for sinus CT scans?

4. On what basis should sinus osteomas be resected?

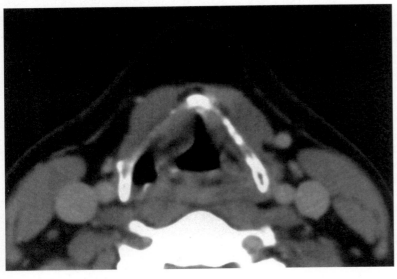 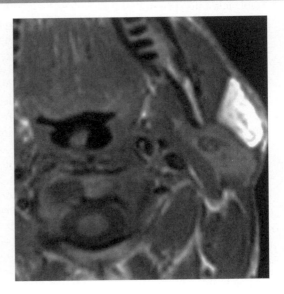

1. What percentage of lipomas occur in the head and neck?

2. Where in the parotid space do lipomas occur?

3. What is the most common site for a lipoma in the head and neck?

4. What are the findings suggestive of a liposarcoma?

Osteoma with a Haller Cell

1. A maxilloethmoidal cell—an ethmoidal air cell extending along the medial and inferior floor of the orbit.

2. It tends to obstruct the maxillary sinus ostium or the infundibulum, predisposing a patient to maxillary or anterior ethmoidal sinusitis.

3. Three percent (peak incidence in the seventh decade of life) based on CT scans, 1% based on plain radiographs.

4. Large osteomas that are accompanied by unrelenting symptoms, that obstruct sinuses, that encompass greater than 50% of the volume of the sinuses, that extend intraorbitally or intracranially, or that grow radiographically should probably be treated surgically.

Reference

Seiden AM, el Hefny YI: Endoscopic trephination for the removal of frontal sinus osteoma, *Otolaryngol Head Neck Surg* 112:607-611, 1995.

Cross-Reference

Neuroradiology: THE REQUISITES, pp 360, 370-371, 390.

Comment

Eighty percent of osteomas occur in the frontal sinuses. The classic history of a frontal osteoma is that of a male patient who, while flying in an airplane on a business trip, has extreme cephalgia caused by the obstruction and superimposed sinus disease. A mucocele may coexist. As tumors, osteomas are very slow growing. Rarely they may perforate into the intracranial space, causing pneumocephalus. More often the presentation is due to headache and sinusitis or mass effect on adjacent structures, be it orbital or intracranial tissue. When osteomas are asymptomatic, it is difficult to decide whether they should be removed (because of their potential growth) or left alone. One must remember the association of Gardner's syndrome: osteomas, colonic polyposis, and soft tissue masses.

   Haller cells should be treated like concha bullosa (aerated middle turbinates). They are considered a normal variant with little import unless they are of such significant size that they obstruct or narrow the ostiomeatal complex, leading to sinusitis. They occur in about one fifth to one fourth of individuals undergoing sinus CT—if you haven't commented on one in the past 20 coronal sinus scans that you've looked at, you probably don't know what they are! Now you do! The surgeon must know about Haller cells because entering these cells to drain sinusitis or relieve ostiomeatal complex narrowing is good medicine. Entering the orbit (the "cell" just superior to the Haller cell) is good business for the lawyers.

Notes

Lipoma in the Superficial Space (Figure on Left) and in the Periparotid Region (Figure on Right)

1. Between 10% and 15% of all soft tissue lipomas.

2. They are equally spread between intraparotid and extraparotid tissue within the parotid space (which is defined by layers of the deep cervical fascia).

3. In the subcutaneous tissues (as in the tissues anterior to the strap muscles in the figure on the left—see it yet?)

4. If one finds nonfatty soft tissue, hemorrhage, or infiltrating margins associated with a lipoma, one had better raise the suggestion of a liposarcoma. Nonetheless, sometimes a liposarcoma exactly simulates a benign lipoma, with no discernible malignant features.

Reference

Kransdorf MJ: Benign soft-tissue tumors in a large referral population: distribution of specific diagnoses by age, sex, and location, *AJR Am J Roentgenol* 164:395-402, 1995.

Cross-Reference

Neuroradiology: THE REQUISITES, pp 421, 435.

Comment

Lipomas have CT attenuation values in the negative 100 to negative 160 HU range. Lipomas are the most common benign soft tissue tumor reported in Kransdorf's series of 18,677 benign mesenchymal masses, with a mean age of 48 and a male predominance. The most common sites are the trunk, head and neck, and lower extremity. If one finds a lipoma with a soft tissue component, one must beware of the dreaded liposarcoma. Liposarcomas are about 1/100th as common as lipomas, but they are the second most common soft tissue sarcoma in adults (children develop rhabdomyosarcomas). Most liposarcomas are found in the retroperitoneum and thigh. In the head and neck most generally occur in the superficial fascia and muscular tissue. In the aerodigestive system the larynx is the most common site for liposarcomas, but chondrosarcomas are the most frequently occurring sarcomas of the larynx. Lymph node metastases from liposarcomas are unheard of. Liposarcomas appear to be due to a translocation between chromosomes 12 and 16 and do not arise from preexisting lipomas.

   Lipomas may respond to changes in weight of the patient. Treatment is usually for cosmetic reasons and consists of surgical removal. Small lipomas may be undetectable clinically and found incidentally on imaging studies. The most common subcutaneous site for a lipoma in the head and neck is the posterior neck.

Notes

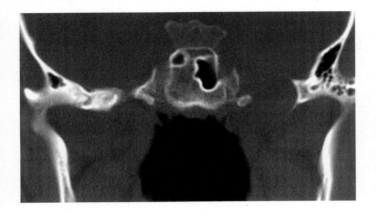 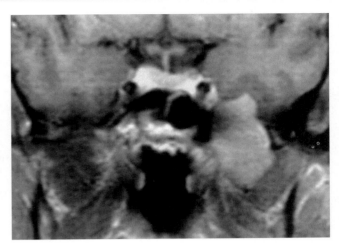

1. Which division of the fifth cranial nerve is most often affected with a schwannoma?
2. What imaging findings in the muscles of mastication can be found with a mandibular nerve schwannoma?
3. Name the exits from the pterygopalatine fossa.
4. Which division of the fifth cranial nerve travels in the pterygopalatine fossa?

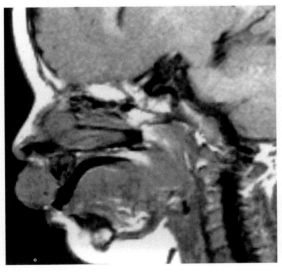 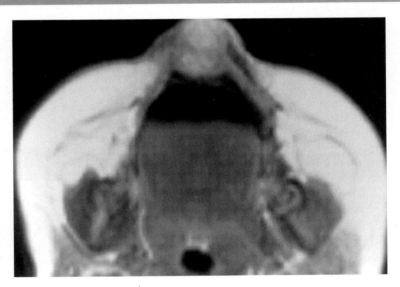

1. What is the most common pediatric head and neck tumor?
2. What MRI findings are typically seen in hemangiomas?
3. What is the most common location for an intramuscular hemangioma of the head and neck?
4. What is the most common deep space of the neck to be involved with a hemangioma?

Fifth Nerve Schwannoma

1. The third division (mandibular nerve).

2. One may see either atrophy or T2W hyperintensity of the muscle and contrast enhancement within the muscle supplied by the schwannoma. One often detects the enhancement and enlargement of the nerve coursing through the muscles or, as in this case, enlargement and enhancement within the foramen ovale.

3. Greater and lesser palatine canals, sphenopalatine foramen, pterygomaxillary fissure, inferior orbital fissure, foramen rotundum, vidian canal, and the cavernous sinus.

4. The second division (maxillary nerve).

Reference

Samii M, Migliori MM, Tatagiba M, Babu R: Surgical treatment of trigeminal schwannomas, *J Neurosurg* 82:711-718, 1995.

Cross-Reference

Neuroradiology: THE REQUISITES, p 328.

Comment

The fifth cranial nerve accounts for the origin of just 1% to 8% of all intracranial schwannomas, being far outnumbered by the seventh and eighth cranial nerves. Multiple schwannomas in concert with neurofibromatosis type 2 account for about one third of patients with trigeminal schwannomas. Blurred vision, headache, facial numbness, paresthesias, and pain usually are the patient's first complaints. Muscle weakness may be present. I have reported and others have confirmed high T2W signal intensity, atrophy, and/or gadolinium enhancement of the muscles of mastication when dealing with a neurogenic tumor that affects the third division of the trigeminal nerve. I have not seen the same with a meningioma, a factor one may want to use in the evidence to support a schwannoma over a meningioma of the trigeminal nerve. One must also remember that meningiomas encase and narrow blood vessels and are more dense on unenhanced CT than schwannomas. On enhanced MRI, intracranial meningiomas sport a dural tail, a finding that is incredibly rare with schwannomas. One must be careful, however, because the dura of Meckel's cave where the trigeminal ganglion resides may show mild enhancement even in normal subjects. Knowing the routes of the three divisions of the fifth cranial nerve will help to follow its pathology.

Notes

Hemangioma of Upper Lip

1. Hemangioma.

2. Dark on T1W scans and bright on T2W scans. Present also may be phleboliths, fibrosis, calcification, and hemorrhage within the tumor, which may alter the signal intensity.

3. The masseter muscle.

4. The parotid space.

Reference

Fine MJ, Holliday RA, Roland JT: Clinically unsuspected venous malformations limited to the submandibular triangle: CT findings, *AJNR Am J Neuroradiol* 16:491-494, 1995.

Cross-Reference

Neuroradiology: THE REQUISITES, pp 348, 391, 398.

Comment

Hemangiomas are easily diagnosed clinically. The patient, usually a child, presents with a discolored skin lesion that is compressible, and the differential diagnosis includes a capillary or cavernous hemangioma, a true arteriovenous malformation, capillary malformations, and lymphohemangiomas. Hemangiomas of childhood rarely necessitate treatment because they often involute by adolescence. Seventy percent of hemangiomas resolve on their own, and 50% have an associated skin "hemangioma." Noninvoluting cavernous hemangiomas of the head and neck have recently been reclassified as *venous vascular malformations.* They are not neoplasms.

When hemangiomas are disfiguring, medical and laser therapy may be attempted; rarely they may be removed surgically. If the lesion occurs deep to the skin, the diagnosis may not be as clear-cut because its reddish hue will not be evident. Operating on these lesions without the prior knowledge that they may be highly vascular could present a surgical nightmare. In general the masses are very bright on T2W MRI and enhance dramatically on CT and MRI with contrast. The major distinction between these tumors and the congenital vascular malformations is that the latter do not involute and may actually grow with time, hormonal influences, infection, thromboses, and/or trauma. Capillary hemangiomas may occur superficially in the skin around the nose, in the nasal bones, on the turbinates, or in the nasal vault along the anterior nasal septum (in Kiesselbach's triangle), where they are seen as well-circumscribed, intensely enhancing masses with bony remodeling. Phleboliths are more characteristic of cavernous hemangiomas.

Notes

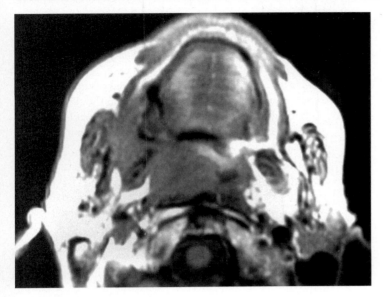

1. What part of the aerodigestive system includes the retromolar trigone?

2. What part of the aerodigestive system includes the hard palate? The soft palate?

3. What bony structures are often resected with a lesion of the retromolar trigone?

4. What are the implications of marrow signal abnormality in the mandible and maxilla of this patient?

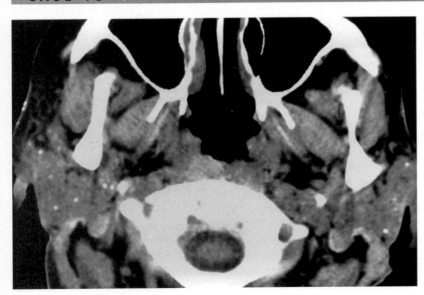

1. Why do calculi occur more commonly in the submandibular gland than in the parotid gland?

2. What disease processes predispose a patient to parotid sialolithiasis?

3. What is the incidence of multiple salivary stones?

4. Nonpainful enlargement of the parotid glands (sialosis) can be seen with what states?

Cancer of the Retromolar Trigone, Palate, and Tonsil

1. The oral cavity.

2. The oral cavity includes the hard palate, but the oropharynx includes the soft palate.

3. The maxillary tuberosity and ascending ramus of the mandible.

4. This MRI finding is highly sensitive but only 75% specific for tumoral infiltration—inflammation, infection, osteoradionecrosis, and fibrosis may simulate neoplastic invasion.

Reference

Unger JM: The oral cavity and tongue: magnetic resonance imaging, *Radiology* 155:151-153, 1985.

Cross-Reference

Neuroradiology: THE REQUISITES, pp 390-393.

Comment

The retromolar trigone is a critical site for squamous cell carcinoma. The retromolar trigone is located behind the maxillary tuberosity and the ascending ramus of the mandible. It usually contains fat and nerves. Because it sits at the junction of the maxilla and the mandible, cancers there often invade one or both of these bony structures. The nearby pterygoid muscles are also fair game for cancers in this region, and invasion is common. A retromolar trigonal cancer may also ascend or spread along the pterygomandibular raphe, which passes by the pterygopalatine fossa. From this location, the tumor may infiltrate the branches of the second division of the fifth cranial nerve. Perineural growth of tumor may direct the tumor into the orbit, the infratemporal fossa, the cavernous sinus, or the middle cranial fossa. One minor salivary gland malignancy, adenoid cystic carcinoma, is notorious for just such spread and may provide an excellent anatomy lesson of the maxillary nerve to the nascent head and neck radiologist. Thus a tumor of the retromolar trigone may necessitate resection of the maxilla, mandible, orbit, temporal bone, and masticator space. Furthermore, the site is not readily approachable surgically, even for a limited resection, and the mandible often has to be rotated laterally for access to the tumor. The "commando" operation is often performed for retromolar trigonal cancers and consists of hemimandibulectomy with resection of the pterygoid and masseter muscles, with an ipsilateral neck dissection. Nodal spread is usually to levels one (submandibular-submental nodes) and two (high jugular nodes above the hyoid bone).

Notes

Parotid Sialolithiasis

1. The submandibular gland saliva is more alkaline (making calcium phosphate and calcium oxalate more likely to precipitate), more mucinous, and thicker. The flow of saliva in the submandibular duct is directed superiorly, causing stasis to occur more frequently in the submandibular duct (Wharton's duct). Wharton's duct is more likely to be traumatized and has a wider diameter than Stensen's duct.

2. Sarcoidosis, Sjögren's disease, and hyperparathyroidism. A strictured duct may lead to stone formation, and stones may lead to strictures—a vicious cycle.

3. Twenty-five percent.

4. Obesity, alcoholism, diabetes, hypothyroidism, malnutrition, cirrhosis, and post partum. Some drugs will also do this.

Reference

Levy DM, ReMine WH, Devine KD: Salivary gland calculi, *JAMA* 181:1115-1119, 1962.

Cross-Reference

Neuroradiology: THE REQUISITES, p 417.

Comment

Sublingual and minor salivary gland calculi are distinctly uncommon. One should exclude calcifications in lymph nodes, tonsils, and vessels before suggesting calculi in these glands. The need for sialography to diagnose calculi is rare these days—unenhanced CT can detect most calculi reliably even if their density is minimally different from surrounding tissue. Enhancing vessels may simulate calculi, so unenhanced scans are best. Most submandibular calculi appear within the duct rather than in the glandular parenchyma. Focal masslike firmness of the submandibular glands caused by chronic sialadenitis from calculus disease (Kuttner tumor) may simulate neoplasms. The pain and swelling of the gland affected with a calculus increases with eating. The closer the calculus is to the duct orifice, the easier the treatment—which may be managed with manual manipulation or surgical excision. Stones within the glandular parenchyma, as in this case, may necessitate glandular removal if the symptoms are such that the patient cannot tolerate the condition. Bilateral intraglandular sialolithiasis is problematic in that bilateral glandular removal may lead to a permanently dry mouth, which is uncomfortable for the patient and may also lead to dental caries.

Notes

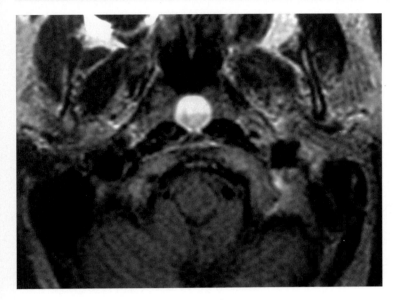

1. What is the likely cause of this lesion?

2. What does the differential diagnosis of a Tornwaldt cyst include?

3. What are the stereotypical signal intensity characteristics of a Tornwaldt cyst?

4. If one finds calcification or nodular contrast enhancement associated with a cystic lesion of the nasopharynx, what should be included in the differential diagnosis?

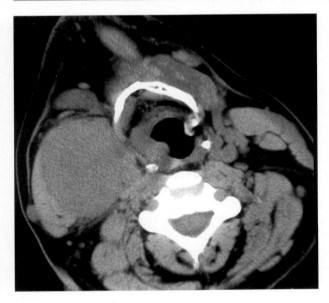

1. What is the typical appearance of lymphomatous cervical adenopathy?

2. Can lymphomatous lymph nodes enhance dramatically?

3. What is the typical histology of lymphoma in the neck?

4. When there is squamous cell carcinoma in a lymph node in the neck without a primary tumor immediately evident, where do most of the primary tumors reside?

T(h)ornwaldt Cyst

1. Retraction of the nasopharyngeal mucosa as the notochord ascends into the clivus and cervical spinal column, causing encystment.

2. Mucous retention cyst, minor salivary gland neoplasms, and serous cyst.

3. High signal intensity on both T1W and T2W scanning.

4. A nasopharyngeal craniopharyngioma, synovial sarcoma, and teratoma.

Reference

Weissmann JL: Thornwaldt cysts, *Am J Otolaryngol* 13:381-385, 1992.

Cross-Reference

Neuroradiology: THE REQUISITES, pp 378-379.

Comment

Tornwaldt (or Thornwaldt) cysts occur as the pharyngeal bursa ectoderm retracts with the notochord into the clivus. The bursa is above the superior pharyngeal constrictor muscle and between the longus muscles. Tornwaldt cysts occur in 3% of healthy adults. Although most are asymptomatic, one may find patients complaining of occipital pain, purulent nasal discharge, nasal obstruction, halitosis, ear fullness, or odynophagia. If the cyst becomes infected it can lead to prevertebral (longus capitis) muscle spasm associated with a foul-smelling discharge. Most Tornwaldt cysts are bright on T1W scans, presumably because of high protein content. These entities have become increasingly well known to radiologists since the advent of MRI. On CT the lesions are of low density and are seen in the midline. Distinguishing a Tornwaldt cyst from a mucous retention cyst, or identifying small Tornwaldt cysts within adenoidal hypertrophy, is much more difficult on CT. Treatment may be benign neglect (nearly all cases), incision, marsupialization, or full extirpation of the cyst. Surgical treatment is reserved for the chronically infected painful cysts.

Gustav Ludwig Tornwaldt lived from 1843 to 1910. Controversy over how he spelled his last name reigns in head and neck radiology circles.

Notes

Lymphoma in Cervical Nodes

1. Large round lymph nodes without necrosis.

2. Yes, particularly in the angiofollicular variety of lymphoma.

3. One can have Hodgkin's disease (HD), which usually affects the supraclavicular lymph nodes, or one can have non-Hodgkin's lymphoma (NHL) (diffuse histiocytic lymphoma), which may affect the lymphoid tissue of the tonsils and adenoids, as well as cervical lymph nodes.

4. The nasopharynx, tonsils, pyriform sinus, or base of the tongue in the head and neck. Breast or lung cancers may be the remote culprits.

Reference

DePena CA, Van Tassel P, Lee YY: Lymphoma of the head and neck, *Radiol Clin North Am* 28:723-744, 1990.

Cross-Reference

Neuroradiology: THE REQUISITES, pp 186, 403-408.

Comment

The most common cause of a neck mass in a young adult patient is cervical adenopathy, and the malignancy to be considered is lymphoma. Nodal necrosis is distinctly uncommon in patients with HD and is seen only a little bit more frequently in those with NHL. The submental, retropharyngeal, submandibular, internal jugular, supraclavicular, and spinal accessory chains are frequently involved with lymphoma. Nearly three quarters of patients with HD present with a neck node, but concurrent disease in the chest is not uncommon. NHL affects extranodal neck tissue (Waldeyer's ring) more frequently than HD, and around 50% of cases with nodal disease have systemic dissemination. Isolated nodal disease is more characteristic of HD than NHL, whereas isolated extranodal manifestations are the hallmark of NHL. Lymphoma accounts for 10% to 15% of malignancies of the orbit, 8% in the paranasal sinuses, 5% in the tonsils, less than 1% in the salivary glands, 2% in the thyroid gland, and less than 5% in the soft tissues.

In a patient with a squamous cell carcinoma neck node and no apparent primary tumor on clinical and endoscopic evaluation, imaging elucidates the primary tumor in many cases. For those cases in which the primary tumor is not present somewhere in the upper aerodigestive system locations listed in Answer 4, one should consider the thyroid gland, the breast, the lungs, and the esophagus as potential primary sites. Positron emission tomography (PET) may be of some benefit in searching for an occult primary tumor—it has been said that the PET scan finds the aerodigestive system primary tumor 25% of the time.

Notes

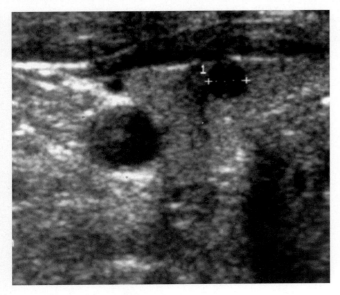

1. How do hemorrhagic cysts of the thyroid gland look?

2. If a cyst has a mural nodule, what is the rate of malignancy?

3. Are most thyroid cancers isoechoic or hypoechoic to normal thyroid tissue?

4. What is the chance that a thyroid mass with an echopenic halo is benign rather than malignant?

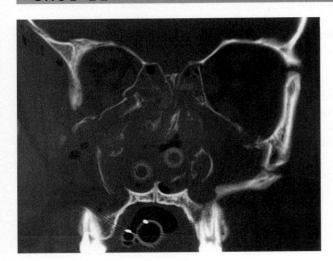

1. What structures are invariably fractured with Le Fort fractures?

2. Is the orbital floor or rim classically fractured with Le Fort II fractures?

3. In which type of Le Fort fracture is the lateral orbit fractured?

4. In which types of Le Fort fracture is the medial orbital wall fractured?

CASE 21

Benign Thyroid Cyst on Ultrasound

1. Hypoechoic (not anechoic).

2. Eleven percent to 14%.

3. Hypoechoic (63%).

4. With an echopenic ring a lesion is over 12 times more likely to be benign than malignant.

Reference
Gooding GA: Sonography of the thyroid and parathyroid, *Radiol Clin North Am* 31:967-989, 1993.

Cross-Reference
Neuroradiology: THE REQUISITES, pp 438-441.

Comment
Pure cysts are almost never malignancies. Mixed cystic and solid lesions are malignant in 11% of cases. If the mass is hyperechoic, one can bet it will be benign in 96% of cases, but an isoechoic mass is malignant in 26%. Therefore a purely cystic lesion and a hyperechoic lesion on ultrasound bode well for the patient. A hypoechoic or isoechoic mass must be investigated further. On ultrasound, the other features that might suggest a malignancy include ill-defined borders and microcalcifications. Well-defined borders, a complete echopenic halo around a lesion, and eggshell calcifications increase the odds that it is a benign process.

Of the different malignancies, the ones that are most commonly hypoechoic are lymphomas and anaplastic carcinomas. Of the ones most commonly isoechoic, the follicular carcinomas and medullary carcinomas stand out. Papillary carcinoma can go both ways. Sharp margins are seen in one third of malignancies.

Pure cysts of the thyroid gland may be seen with colloid cysts, with degeneration of adenomas, and within multinodular goiters.

Notes

CASE 22

Le Fort Fractures

1. The pterygoid plates.

2. Rim.

3. III.

4. II and III.

Reference
Kreipke DL, Moss JJ, Franco JM, Maves MD, Smith DJ: Computed tomography and thin-section tomography in facial trauma, *AJNR Am J Neuroradiol* 5:185-189, 1984.

Cross-Reference
Neuroradiology: THE REQUISITES, pp 166-167.

Comment
I tend to describe fractures by their location rather than by their eponyms, but this may be because I am forgetful with names and can never remember classifications. Suffice it to say, Le Fort I fractures predominantly involve the lower maxilla and do not usually involve the orbits, whereas Le Fort II fractures affect the inferior and medial orbits. Le Fort III fractures cross from lateral orbit to medial orbit and are the fracture constellations in which "craniofacial dissociation" may occur. That is, the facial bones inferiorly are relatively disconnected from the skull above. Common to all of these fractures is extension across the pterygoid plates. Trimalar fractures affect the attachments of the zygoma to the maxilla, the frontal bone, and the sphenoid bones. They create a lateral divot out of the side of the face, dissociating the lateral orbit, zygoma, and lateral edge of the maxilla from the rest of the face.

Looking at the images provided, one would say that this patient has evidence of Le Fort II and III fractures on the left and probably a Le Fort II fracture on the right. Obviously there are many more fractures seen, predominantly involving the sinonasal cavity and septum. The tubes in the nose and mouth are for nasogastric and endotracheal intubations.

Notes

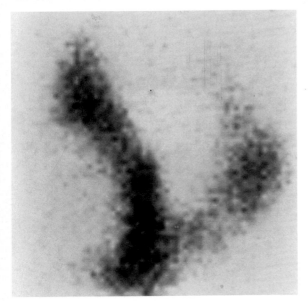

1. What are the two most common agents used to evaluate the thyroid gland in nuclear medicine studies?
2. What are the different energies of these agents?
3. How often is a solitary cold nodule malignant?
4. What increases that risk?

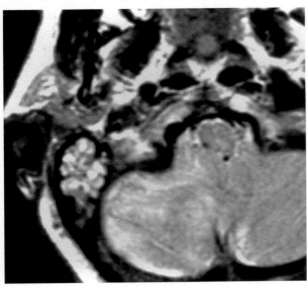 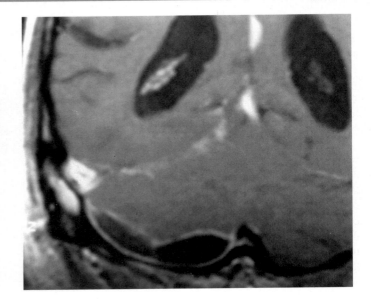

1. Define coalescent mastoiditis.
2. Why do subperiosteal abscesses of the mastoid antrum occur in a posterior auricular location?
3. What intracranial complications are evident on this patient's films?
4. Which dural sinus is most closely apposed to the mastoid air cells?

Cold Nodule on Thyroid Scintigraphy

1. Iodine-123 and technetium Tc 99m pertechnetate.

2. Iodine-123 has 159 keV photons, and ^{99m}Tc pertechnetate produces 140 keV photons.

3. Approximately 15% of the time.

4. Having been exposed to radiation, being younger than 20 or older than 60, being male, having a family history of thyroid cancers, or having multiple endocrine neoplasia syndrome.

Reference

Loevner LA: Imaging of the thyroid gland, *Semin Ultrasound CT MR* 17:539-562, 1996.

Cross-Reference

Neuroradiology: THE REQUISITES, p 440.

Comment

The work-up of any solitary cold nodule should probably include fine needle aspiration, particularly for the at-risk groups listed above. Some physicians (including myself) believe that the most cost-effective way to manage a palpable thyroid mass is either to perform an ultrasound (to exclude a pure cyst or multinodular goiter) or to skip that step and go right to fine needle aspiration and cytology. Too often the imaging findings are nonspecific and cannot exclude a cancer (since thyroid cancers can look like anything), so why not just sample the tissue? Thyroid glands are the "breasts" of the head and neck surgeon—one aspirates many benign lesions to find a single malignancy.

Irradiation for thymic enlargement, acne, tinea capitis, and adenoidal hypertrophy in the 1930s and 1940s induced a spike in thyroid carcinoma 30 to 40 years later. Interestingly, the increased incidence of thyroid cancers in irradiated individuals occurred only in those who had received up to a dose of 1500 rad. Above that, one actually sees a drop in incidence of thyroid cancer (a good thing too for all of those patients with head and neck squamous cell carcinoma who receive primary or postoperative radiation therapy). In my practice there seems to have been a shift recently to older individuals developing anaplastic carcinoma. Lymphoma of the thyroid gland is also seen more commonly now, usually in association with Hashimoto's thyroiditis. One should remember also that medullary carcinoma is the thyroid malignancy that is associated with pheochromocytomas, parathyroid hyperplasia, and marfanoid facies in multiple endocrine neoplasia type II. The anaplastic and medullary carcinomas of the thyroid gland have a much worse prognosis than the papillary or follicular types. The papillary or follicular types have a disease-related mortality under 20%.

Notes

Mastoiditis with Epidural Abscess

1. An infection of the mastoid air cell in which there is erosion of mastoid septa, creating an inflammatory mass with associated osteomyelitis of the bone.

2. There is thin bone in this location, allowing loculation of inflammatory debris within *Macewen's triangle.*

3. Epidural abscess, meningitis, and probable partial transverse sinus thrombosis.

4. Sigmoid sinus.

Reference

Holliday RA, Reede DL: MRI of mastoid and middle ear disease, *Radiol Clin North Am* 27:283-299, 1989.

Cross-Reference

Neuroradiology: THE REQUISITES, pp 172-173, 343, 479.

Comment

Mastoid air cell aeration can be quite variable, and in children who suffer from chronic otitis media the mastoid may be underpneumatized. This leads to unusual signal intensities on MRI because the presence of marrow fat in the bone causes increased signal intensity on T1W and fast T2W scans, giving the semblance of chronic fluid accumulation in some cases. Most cases of mastoiditis arise in association with middle ear disease, which in turn may be secondary to malfunction or obstruction of the eustachian tube. The potential complications of mastoiditis are protean, as demonstrated in this case. Sinus thromboses or thrombophlebitis may be present, leading to venous infarctions and/or intraparenchymal abscesses. A Bezold's abscess refers to perforation of the mastoid antrum with extension of the inflammatory mass into the soft tissues of the neck. *Pneumococcus* and *Haemophilus influenzae* are the most common organisms causing otomastoiditis.

CT remains the most effective way to study the middle ear and mastoid air cells for inflammatory disease. MRI was used in this case to examine the intracranial complications from the known otomastoiditis.

Notes

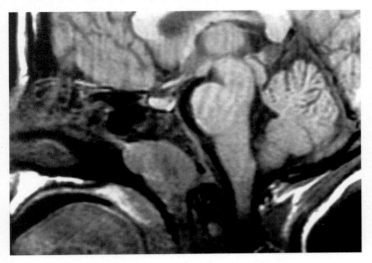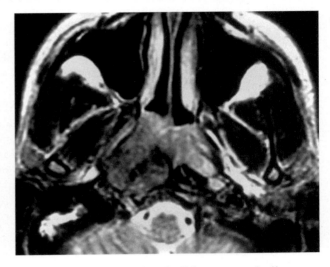

1. Which is more likely to occur—a mucosal lesion of the nasopharynx growing into the skull base, or a skull base tumor growing into the nasopharynx?

2. Through what orifices might this lesion spread into the intracranial compartment?

3. What are the histologic subtypes of nasopharyngeal carcinoma?

4. Name predisposing factors for nasopharyngeal carcinomas.

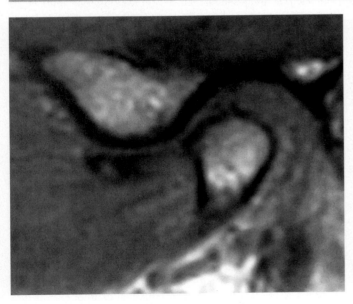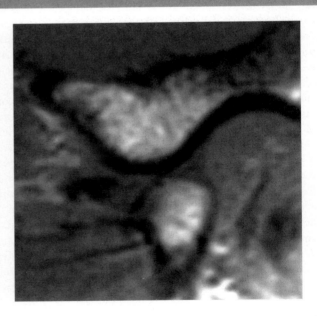

1. Describe the findings in this case.

2. What is the significance of medial or lateral subluxation of the meniscus of the temporomandibular joint?

3. What is a "stuck disk"?

4. What percentage of asymptomatic volunteers have anterior dislocation of their menisci?

CASE 25

Nasopharyngeal Carcinoma

1. A nasopharynx cancer growing into the skull base.

2. Through the foramen ovale (via the third division of the fifth cranial nerve), along the foramen rotundum (via the second division of the fifth cranial nerve), or via the jugular foramen, hypoglossal canal, or foramen lacerum.

3. They include keratinizing squamous cell carcinomas, non-keratinizing carcinomas, and undifferentiated carcinomas. Within the undifferentiated category, lymphoepitheliomas are one of the most common varieties of tumors and show a particularly favorable response to radiation therapy.

4. EBV exposure, Southeast Asian parentage, and specific HLA subtypes in the Asian populations. Smoking and alcohol use do not appear to be significant risk factors.

Reference

Chong VFH, Fan Y-F: Detection of recurrent nasopharyngeal carcinoma: MR imaging versus CT, *Radiology* 202:463-470, 1997.

Cross-Reference

Neuroradiology: THE REQUISITES, p 430.

Comment

The incidence of nasopharyngeal carcinoma in the native or immigrant Asian population is about 20 times greater than in the white U.S. population. EBV polymerase chain reaction positivity is found in the nonkeratinizing carcinomas and undifferentiated carcinomas but not in the keratinizing squamous cell tumors and adenocarcinomas. Nasopharyngeal carcinoma is not treated surgically—a cure relies on radiation therapy and/or chemotherapy. Once disease has gone intracranially or outside the nasopharynx, the prognosis is poor, mainly because of the higher incidence of hematogenous metastases and poor local control rates. After radiotherapy (and chemotherapy) there is often fibrotic change that resembles persistent tumor. One should rely on the presence of a defined mass and enhancing focal tissue rather than mucosal asymmetry to suggest persistent or recurrent disease. Lobulation is bad, smoothness is good. MRI has been shown to be superior to CT for both the initial and the follow-up evaluations of nasopharyngeal carcinoma. Because nasopharyngeal tumors often burrow submucosally, imaging and nasopharyngoscopy play complementary roles. For spread to the lymph nodes (retropharyngeal ones in 50%), imaging is superior to clinical evaluation. The mechanism of spread through the skull base may be through the fascial planes and bone or via perineural extension.

Notes

CASE 26

Anterior Dislocation without Recapture of the Meniscus of the Temporomandibular Joint

1. Anterior dislocation on closed mouth view (figure on left) without recapture on open mouth view (figure on right), degenerative beaking of the mandibular condyle, and minimal erosion of the condylar head.

2. With either rotational or sideways dislocation of the disk, there is a reduced chance of reduction in the open mouth view or with conservative treatment.

3. A meniscus that does not move between the open and closed mouth positions, usually caused by fibrotic adhesions.

4. Fifteen percent to 30%.

Reference

Brooks SL, Westesson PL: Temporomandibular joint: value of coronal MR images, *Radiology* 188:317-321, 1993.

Cross-Reference

Neuroradiology: THE REQUISITES, pp 426-427.

Comment

Anterior displacement of the meniscus is believed to be due to an imbalance between the anterior pull of the tendon of the lateral pterygoid muscle and the retraction afforded by the elastic fibers of the bilaminar zone that insert on the posterior band of the meniscus. Anterior dislocations of the meniscus are far and away the most common types of displacement and are best seen on sagittal closed and open mouth MRI scans. The posterior edge of the meniscus should be within 10 degrees of vertical with the mandibular condyle.

Although most radiologists rely on the sagittal scans to diagnose meniscal displacement, the medial or lateral subluxation of the disk is better visualized on direct coronal scans. It has been estimated that in 25% to 33% of cases there is a mediolateral component of disk displacement with or without the anterior dislocation. Pure (without an anterior component) sideways medial or lateral disk displacements occur in about 10% of cases. Although most radiologists are busy enough just trying to identify the disk, the demonstration of this extra sideways component is important because it portends a worse prognosis with respect to standard therapies (splinting, behavioral modifications) for temporomandibular joint disease. Coronal scans add information to the sagittal study in 13% of cases and confirm suspected mediolateral components of disk displacement in another 13%. I like them. One should also make sure that the meniscus moves on jaw opening. "Stuck disks," which are immobile between open and closed mouth views, are usually symptomatic.

Notes

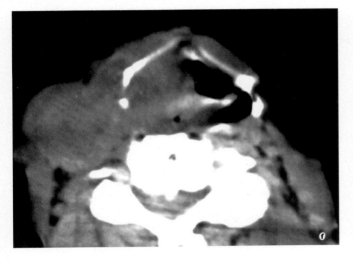
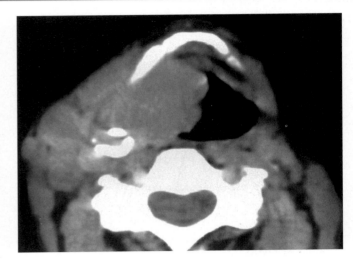

1. Localize this lesion.

2. Of primary sites of head and neck cancer, which is the most common to directly encase the carotid artery?

3. Define the subsites of the hypopharynx.

4. If a fistula occurs to the pyriform sinus, what should one consider?

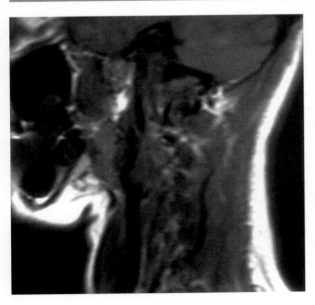
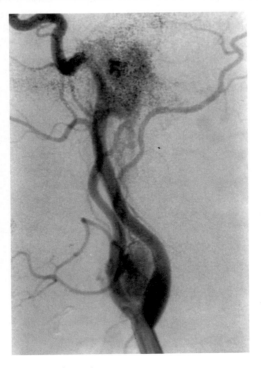

1. What are the classic locations of these lesions in the head and neck?

2. How can one make a definitive diagnosis of paraganglioma as opposed to a schwannoma in these locations?

3. How often are paragangliomas multiple?

4. What precautions should be taken before embolization of paragangliomas?

Hypopharyngeal Squamous Cell Carcinoma

1. It is centered in the right pyriform sinus and grows extrapharyngeally into the soft tissues of the neck. Nodes are also present.

2. The pyriform sinus.

3. The pyriform sinus, the postcricoid region, and the posterior pharyngeal wall from the pharyngoepiglottic fold to the level of the cricoarytenoid joints.

4. Malignancy versus a tract from a branchial cleft fistula.

Reference

Zbaren P, Egger C: Growth patterns of pyriform sinus cancer, *Laryngoscope* 107:511-518, 1997.

Cross-Reference

Neuroradiology: THE REQUISITES, pp 393-394.

Comment

By combining imaging with clinical evaluation of hypopharyngeal cancers, one increases the accuracy of TNM (primary *T*umor, *N*odes, *M*etastatic site) staging from 48% (clinical alone) to 92% (clinical and imaging). Cartilage invasion and nodal disease are the areas where imaging most commonly helps, but extrapharyngeal extension is also well depicted with imaging. Furthermore, surgical/therapeutic planning for patients is altered if and when imaging demonstrates carotid artery, vertebral artery, posterior musculature, preepiglottic fat, paraglottic space, or bony invasion. MRI is superior to CT on many of these issues but necessitates good technique and experienced interpretation. One can get away with a schlock CT of the neck, but a bad MRI of the neck often is worthless.

Hypopharyngeal carcinoma affects the paraglottic tissues more commonly than the contralateral hypopharynx, the thyroid cartilage, and the preepiglottic fat—in that order. A propensity for perineural extension explains the frequent treatment failures with this cancer. Plus, patients with cancers in this location are rarely diagnosed when under stage T2. Fixation of the hemilarynx occurs in about 80% of cases (T3 cancer), often because of invasion of the paraglottic tissues or intrinsic muscles of the laryngeal vocal cords more so than invasion of the cricoarytenoid joints. Nodal metastases are found in 75% of pyriform sinus cancers. Voice conservation therapy is often inadequate treatment of hypopharyngeal cancers because of the frequent cartilage invasion, cord fixation, bilateral involvement, and extensive paraglottic spread.

Notes

Carotid Body and Glomus Jugulare Lesions

1. In the jugular foramen, along the vagus nerve, in the tympanic cavity, and at the carotid bifurcation.

2. Contrast-enhanced dynamic MRI studies are most specific in diagnosing paragangliomas. One finds rapid uptake of contrast in the lesion in the first 60 seconds after contrast administration, punctuated by a slight dip in signal intensity at about 20 to 40 seconds, followed by a second phase of signal increase.

3. Approximately 3% to 5% of the time, but there are familial forms of the disease in which multiplicity is as high as 20% to 30%.

4. Because they may secrete norepinephrine, serotonin, dopamine, or other vasoactive substances, one should check urinary catecholamines. If they are elevated, α-blockers and/or β-blockers administered at the time of angiography may prevent a hypertensive crisis.

Reference

Vogl TJ, Juergens M, Balzer JO, Mack MG, Bergman C, Grevers G, Lissner J, Felix R: Glomus tumors of the skull base: combined use of MR angiography and spin-echo imaging, *Radiology* 192:103-110, 1994.

Cross-Reference

Neuroradiology: THE REQUISITES, pp 344, 346.

Comment

The jugular bulb is a difficult area to evaluate because of its turbulent venous flow, which can cause unusual signal intensity and enhancement patterns. With a normal jugular vein or a high riding one, one may see soft tissue intensity in the bulb on T1W scans that is bright on T2W scans and enhances avidly. These intensity patterns exactly simulate a glomus jugulare. How can turbulent flow in the bulb and a glomus jugulare be distinguished? Hopefully one will see phase ghosting in the normally flowing bulb, but sometimes one may have to do a flow sensitive MR venogram to sort this out.

Dynamic MRI shows a dip in the dynamic curve at the 20 to 40 second mark after administration of contrast agents that is characteristic of the sigmoid sinus, jugular bulb, and paragangliomas. No drop-out effect is seen with schwannomas, meningiomas, or carcinomas, which instead show a gradual decline in intensity. One should look for the "salt and pepper" internal architecture of glomus tumors but not rely on it too heavily—small tumors (under 2 cm) may look homogeneous, and some lesions never show the classic flow voids of the "pepper."

Notes

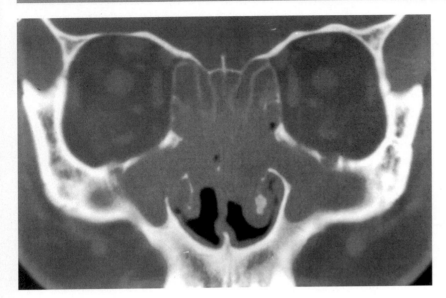

1. What is the success rate of functional endoscopic sinus surgery in patients with sinonasal polyposis treated with total ethmoidectomy?

2. What is the incidence of abnormalities in the paranasal sinuses (i.e., mucosal thickening, air-fluid levels, polypoid excrescences) on CT scans of children with no clinical signs and symptoms of sinusitis?

3. Describe the appearance of the inflammatory pseudotumor of the paranasal sinuses.

4. Contrast the differential diagnoses of patients who have (1) a solitary discrete area of increased density (calcification), (2) multiple discrete areas of increased density, and (3) diffuse areas of increased density within their sinuses.

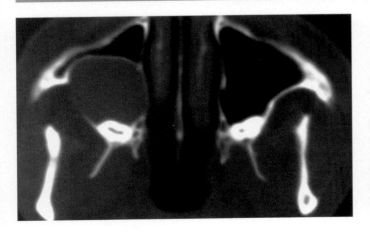 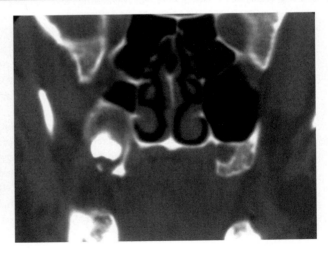

1. What is the sine qua non of dentigerous cysts?

2. What neoplasms are also associated with unerupted teeth?

3. What lesions are associated with impacted teeth?

4. What odontogenic lesions are associated with nonvital teeth?

Sinonasal Polyposis

1. Symptomatic improvement is reported in 80% of cases.

2. Approximately 40%.

3. It is found in the maxillary sinus and is associated with either focal bone erosion, bony remodeling, or bony sclerosis with or without extension into the orbit. Intermediate signal intensity is noted on MRI.

4. A solitary discrete area of increased density is most likely caused by an inflammatory lesion, whereas multifocal calcifications or densities are just as likely to be found in a tumor as in an inflammatory lesion. Diffuse increased density is usually seen in fibroosseous benign bony lesions unless it is an aggressive erosive process, in which case it may be a chondro- or osteosarcoma.

Reference

Phillips CD, Platts-Mills TA: Chronic sinusitis: relationship between CT findings and clinical history of asthma, allergy, eosinophilia, and infection, *AJR Am J Roentgenol* 164:185-188, 1996.

Cross-Reference

Neuroradiology: THE REQUISITES, p 369.

Comment

Chronic sinusitis may be associated with asthma, polyps, eosinophilia, cystic fibrosis, Kartagener's syndrome, and allergies. Aspirin sensitivity may also be a component of the illness. Alternatively, chronic sinusitis may be due to anatomic variations in sinonasal and ostiomeatal anatomy that predispose the ostia to occlusions. Mucoperiosteal thickening, mucous retention cysts, osteitis, and polypoid mucosa may be evident on CT scans.

Polyps are commonly seen in patients with Churg-Strauss syndrome, allergic fungal sinusitis, cilia dyskinetic (Kartagener's) syndrome, and Young's syndrome. Nasal polyps are more common in patients with nonallergic asthma than in those with allergic asthma.

I perform scans in the coronal plane with bone windows and bone algorithms only but put a caveat in reports that the exam is inadequate to evaluate intraorbital and intracranial manifestations of disease. The trade-off is that patients are charged just a little over twice the price of plain films for this study. If complications of sinusitis are suspected, then axial, coronal bone, and soft tissue windows and algorithms are performed, but the patient is charged a hefty rate.

I suggest the diagnosis of polyps whenever I see mass effect or ostial widening associated with sinonasal opacification. I use the term *polypoid mucosal thickening* whenever I see rounded excrescences off the mucosal surface. It seems to serve me well.

Notes

Dentigerous Cyst

1. A cyst associated with an unerupted tooth.

2. Ameloblastomas.

3. Adenomatoid odontogenic tumors and Pindborg tumors.

4. Radicular cysts, Garré's sclerosing osteomyelitis, and cementomas.

Reference

Han MH, Chang KH, Lee CH, Na DG, Yeon KM, Han MC: Cystic expansile masses of the maxilla: differential diagnosis with CT and MR, *AJNR Am J Neuroradiol* 16:333-338, 1995.

Cross-Reference

Neuroradiology: THE REQUISITES, pp 388-389.

Comment

When dealing with a cyst of the maxilla, one of the fundamental questions to be answered is, "Did the lesion come from the tooth or the maxillary sinus?" In most cases, observing the pattern of bony remodeling leads to a definitive answer. Upward bowing of the floor of the antrum suggests odontogenic origin, even if that bone is thinned. Bony septa between lesions and antral walls suggest mucoceles. Obviously, CT is better than MRI for making these distinctions, and plain films may also be very useful.

Dentigerous cysts are usually unilocular, well demarcated, expansile, associated with an unerupted tooth, and occur most commonly in the mandible. A predilection for the upper and lower third molars is seen. In children, the premolars seem to be affected. Treatment necessitates removal of both the cyst and the unerupted tooth. Patients with various forms of mucopolysaccharidoses have a predilection for dentigerous cysts. An ameloblastoma may occur in association with a dentigerous cyst. DentaScanning (a CT technique) may be particularly useful in evaluating dental cysts because it nicely demonstrates the relationship of the lesion to the inferior alveolar canal.

Notes

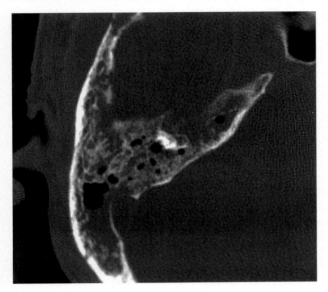

1. What is the most common cause of petrous apicitis?

2. What runs through Dorello's canal?

3. What runs through the inferior petrosal sinus?

4. What is the mechanism by which cholesterol granulomas of the petrous apex form?

CASE 32

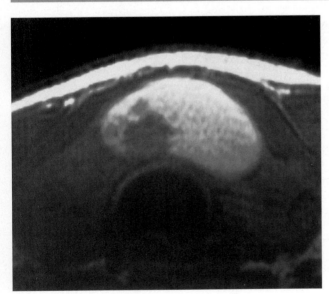

1. What does the differential diagnosis of a hyperintense mass in or around the thyroid gland include?

2. How accurate is cytology in evaluating thyroid lesions?

3. If one sees a diffusely infiltrative lesion of the thyroid gland and surrounding tissues, what does the differential diagnosis include?

4. What is the energy of iodine-131 for treatment of thyroid gland malignancies and imaging of metastases?

CASE 31

Mastoiditis and Erosive Petrous Apicitis

1. Extension of otomastoiditis into the petrous apex. Causative organisms are *Pneumococcus* and *Haemophilus influenzae.*

2. The sixth cranial nerve. (It can be affected by petrous apicitis, as can the fifth cranial nerve.)

3. The sixth cranial nerve.

4. It is thought that there is vascular leakage caused by atmospheric pressure differences in an aerated petrous apex. This causes petechial bleeding, fostering a foreign body reaction and additional exudation of hemorrhagic material into the petrous apex. Ultimately there are cholesterin crystals and hemorrhagic by-products present in an expanded mass in the petrous apex.

Reference
Curtin HD, Som PM: The petrous apex, *Otolaryngol Clin North Am* 28:473-496, 1995.

Cross-Reference
Neuroradiology: THE REQUISITES, p 353.

Comment
Petrous apicitis may occur as a manifestation of middle ear disease because these air cells drain to the middle ear. One must remember that only 30% of individuals have aeration of the petrous apex, and only in these individuals is there the potential for petrous apicitis, cholesterol granulomas, and mucoceles. From the petrous apex, infection may spread to the meninges or to the dural sinuses, making this a precarious location to have an infection. Sinus thromboses, petrous carotid inflammatory pseudoaneurysms, epidural abscesses, and meningitis may complicate severe petrous apicitis. Mucoceles of the petrous apex may have a variety of signal intensities, depending on protein content.

There are some important imaging findings on this CT scan. One should note that there is inflammation and dehiscence of bone right next to the sigmoid sinus groove. Discontinuity of bone also appears to be present anterolaterally and anteromedially near the superior semicircular canal. One should also note extension of opacified air cells anteriorly into the lateral skull of the middle cranial fossa. All of these findings are a "set-up" for meningitis, sinus thrombosis, epidural abscesses, and thrombophlebitis.

Notes

CASE 32

Colloid Cyst and Nodule of the Thyroid Gland

1. Thyroglossal duct cysts and colloid cysts are often bright on T1W scans. Alternatively, one can find hemorrhagic cystadenocarcinomas, teratomas, lipomas, and dermoid tumors, which are hyperintense on T1W scans. Melanoma or thyroid nodal metastases may also be bright.

2. Approximately 90% accurate.

3. Thyroid carcinoma (adenocarcinoma or anaplastic carcinoma), lymphoma, metastatic disease to the thyroid gland, and Riedel's thyroiditis.

4. 364 keV.

Reference
Sanchez RB, vanSonnenberg E, D'Agostino HB, Shank T, Oglevie S, O'Laoide R, Fundell L, Robbins T: Ultrasound-guided biopsy of nonpalpable and difficult to palpate thyroid masses, *J Am Coll Surg* 178:33-37, 1994.

Cross-Reference
Neuroradiology: THE REQUISITES, pp 439-440, 512.

Comment
Palpation or ultrasound-guided aspiration is probably the most economic method for evaluating most asymptomatic thyroid nodules. Why should one bother with nonspecific CT, MRI, ultrasound, or invariably cold nuclear medicine scans to study an enlarging thyroid nodule when one can get a few cells or tissue to make a diagnosis? Diagnostic material is usually obtained in about 85% of cases, and the cytopathologists are correct in 95% of cases in which adequate material is obtained. Complications are vanishingly rare and are usually limited to hematomas. Most people prefer 25-gauge needles to puncture the mass; I tend to get meatier specimens with a 22-gauge needle but would not go larger than that. True biopsies and histologic specimens for thyroid lesions are rarely performed because of the relatively high rate of bleeding induced by the larger cutting needles required for these purposes. It is not uncommon to perform five passes in the thyroid gland during which the cytologist just keeps saying, "Blood. Blood. Blood. Blood. Blood." One should get it right the first time or the odds for doing so seem to be decreased.

The MRIs performed for thyroid masses are not performed for diagnostic purposes but rather to assess for invasion of the trachea, esophagus, or vascular structures once neoplasm has been established. Intrathoracic growth of the lesion is probably better evaluated with CT because the lesion may extend beyond the range of the MRI surface coil.

Notes

34

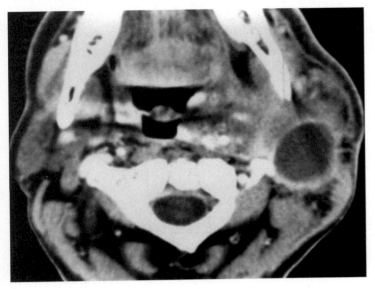

1. What is the most common site of a branchial cleft cyst?

2. Rank the four branchial clefts, from most likely to cause a cyst to least likely.

3. What lines a branchial cleft cyst wall?

4. If a second branchial cleft cyst fistulizes, where does it go?

CASE 34

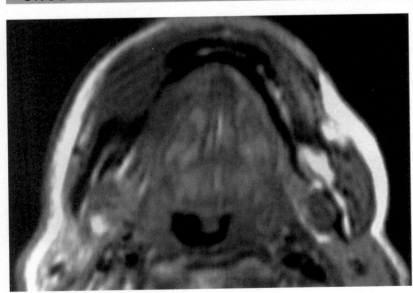

1. What part of the head and neck is the floor of the mouth? What makes up the floor of the mouth?

2. What benign lesions occur in the floor of the mouth?

3. What stage tumor of the floor of the mouth has extrinsic tongue muscle invasion?

4. What is the most common site of oral cavity cancer?

Branchial Cleft Cyst

1. Anterior to the sternocleidomastoid muscle at the level of the carotid bifurcation (angle of the mandible).

2. II > I > IV > III.

3. Respiratory epithelium.

4. To the palatine tonsil.

Reference

Benson MT, Dalen K, Mancuso AA, Kerr HH, Cacciarelli AA, MaFee MF: Congenital anomalies of the branchial apparatus: embryology and pathologic anatomy, *Radiographics* 12:943-960, 1992.

Cross-Reference

Neuroradiology: THE REQUISITES, pp 336, 416.

Comment

This could easily be a necrotic node in a patient with squamous cell carcinoma. The rim is a little thin for that, however, and the mass is very rounded. In a young patient, one would favor an infected branchial cleft cyst. A second branchial anomaly may have its cutaneous fistula at the anterior border of the lower portion of the sternocleidomastoid muscle. It may drain internally (after passing between internal and external carotid arteries) into the tonsillar fossa, after having crossed the parapharyngeal space. This accounts for the rare but possible occurrence of a second branchial cleft cyst in the prestyloid parapharyngeal space. Four types of second branchial cleft cysts are described by Bailey: (I) superficial under platysma, anterior to the sternocleidomastoid muscle, (II) on the great vessels near the angle of the mandible, anterior to the sternocleidomastoid muscle, (III) between the great vessels and the lateral pharyngeal wall (possibly in the parapharyngeal space), and (IV) against the pharyngeal wall near the tonsil. Mimics of second branchial apparatus lesions include venous thromboses, dermoids, neurogenic tumors, eccentric thyroglossal duct cysts, cystic thyroid cancer nodal metastases, and external fluid-filled laryngoceles.

Notes

Oral Cavity Squamous Cell Carcinoma with Mandibular Invasion

1. It is a part of the oral cavity and consists of the mylohyoid muscle and the sublingual space.

2. Ranulas, dermoids, lymphangiomas, thyroglossal duct cysts, and hemangiomas.

3. T4.

4. The lip.

Reference

Mukherji SK, Weeks SM, Castillo M, Yankaskas BC, Krishnan LA, Schiro S: Squamous cell carcinomas that arise in the oral cavity and tongue base: can CT help predict perineural or vascular invasion? *Radiology* 198:157-162, 1996.

Cross-Reference

Neuroradiology: THE REQUISITES, p 393.

Comment

Head and neck surgeons require 2-cm margins around a visible tumor to feel comfortable that they have resected all macro- and microscopic disease. However, they may use the periosteum of the mandible and periorbita of the orbit as a margin, even if it is a "close" one. With floor of mouth cancers, one must be aware of the implications of neurovascular infiltration of the hypoglossal and lingual nerve and lingual artery. There is a greater risk of lymph node metastases, local and nodal recurrences, and death from the tumor when these neurovascular structures of the floor of the mouth and tongue base are infiltrated with tumor. The two nerves and the artery course in the sublingual space, closely related to the styloglossus/hyoglossus complex—if the fat is obliterated between the tumor and this muscle and/or the enhancing vessels, and if irregular margins of the tumor are seen in the sublingual space, one should call infiltration of the neurovascular sheath. Even if it is close, the artery and nerves may end up in the bucket as part of the 2-cm margin. First echelon nodal drainage from the floor of the mouth is to level 1 (submandibular and submental) and level 2 (high jugular chains) nodes.

The findings in this case suggest that the site of origin of this cancer may have been from the buccal (lateral) mucosa of the cheek or the alveolar ridge (tooth sockets). There is a component that extends onto the lingual surface of the mandible and then onto the mylohyoid muscle, but that is smaller than the mandibular and superficial component. The mucosa overlying the mandible is termed the gingiva.

Notes

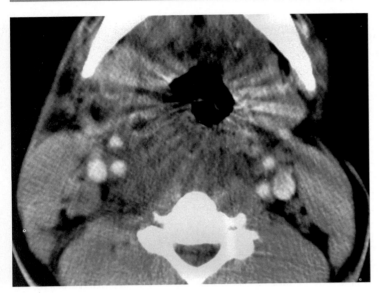

1. Where is this lesion located? What markers separate the lesion from the perivertebral region?
2. From the retropharyngeal space, how can an inflammatory lesion extend inferiorly?
3. What is the usual source of a retropharyngeal abscess?
4. What are complications of peritonsillar abscesses?

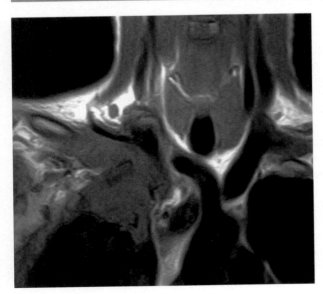

1. What is the most common organ of origin of a Pancoast tumor?
2. What infections may mimic a Pancoast tumor?
3. Why do patients develop brachial plexopathy and Horner's syndrome with these lesions?
4. From what non–lung parenchyma neoplasms can one develop a Pancoast syndrome?

ANSWERS

CASE 35

Retropharyngitis
1. In the pharyngeal mucosa and retropharyngeal space. It involves and is posterior to the mucosa but remains anterior to the longus colli musculature.
2. The retropharyngeal space extends to the midthoracic level. Via the danger space, a retropharyngeal abscess can extend inferiorly to the diaphragm.
3. Pharyngitis, tonsillitis, retropharyngeal adenitis, and/or peritonsillar abscesses.
4. Septic aneurysms, jugular thrombophlebitis, cellulitis, and mediastinitis.

Reference
Ekberg O, Sjoberg S: Neck pain and dysphagia: MRI of retropharyngitis, *J Comput Assist Tomogr* 19:555-558, 1995.

Cross-Reference
Neuroradiology: THE REQUISITES, pp 433-435.

Comment
Retropharyngeal processes usually induce neck pain, limited range of movement of the neck, dysphagia, and odynophagia. The differential diagnosis may include tendonitis of the longus colli muscles (usually associated with calcifications). The retropharyngeal space is bounded anteriorly by the buccopharyngeal membrane and part of the middle layer of the deep cervical fascia, laterally by the alar fascia, and posteriorly by the prevertebral fascia. Some say that the alar and buccopharyngeal fasciae fuse above C3 and below C6, which accounts for the possibility of a localized retropharyngitis between these cervical segments. A reflection of the fascial planes of the retropharyngeal space creates the "danger space." In 9 years of experience with head and neck pathology, I have only seen one case of retropharyngeal pathology pass down to the midthoracic region, presumably spread via the danger space. Nonetheless, it is a pet topic for many head and neck aficionados.

I use displacement of the longus colli–longus capitis complex to distinguish retropharyngeal (anterior to these muscles) from perivertebral (posterior to these muscles) processes. Displacement of the muscles posteriorly implies a pharyngeal or retropharyngeal lesion. This adage may be of particular use when there are massive skull base lesions that have head and neck components. If the lesion arises in bone (a metastasis, chordoma, or sarcoma) it should push the longus complex anteriorly.

Notes

CASE 36

Pancoast Tumor
1. The lung (non–small cell carcinomas).
2. The classic infection involves actinomycosis growing through the chest wall, but nocardia, *Staphylococcus,* blastomycosis, and tuberculosis are all capable of producing a virulent lung apex–chest wall mass.
3. Invasion through the chest wall into the brachial plexus from below and involvement of the cervical stellate ganglion of the sympathetic plexus account for the symptoms associated with a Pancoast tumor.
4. Breast cancer, multiple myeloma, bone metastases, mesothelioma, lymphoma, and Kaposi's sarcoma (in AIDS patients).

Reference
Kuhlman JE, Bouchardy L, Fishman EK, Zerhouni EA: CT and MR imaging evaluation of chest wall disorders, *Radiographics* 14:571-595, 1994.

Cross-Reference
Neuroradiology: THE REQUISITES, pp 435-437.

Comment
In children a neuroblastoma may present with a Pancoast-like configuration. The superior sulcus syndrome may include ipsilateral arm pain in the C8-T2 distribution and atrophy of the hand muscles, in addition to Horner's syndrome and brachial plexopathy. Rib destruction and vertebral body infiltration are not unusual. The lung cancers are usually non–small cell carcinomas. Radiation and surgery combined provide the best outcome. Often patients receive pre- and postoperative irradiation (the latter for patients with incomplete resections). Long-term survival is negligible for those patients with incomplete resection, large adenopathy, or malignant invasion of ribs. Two of the most common sites of postoperative residual tumor with a Pancoast carcinoma are the brachial plexus and the supraaortic vessels. Therefore it behooves the radiologist to be particularly cognizant in mentioning tumor spread to and around these sites. The patient shown here clearly has disease encasing vascular structures and, if the extent of the tumor posteriorly is analogous to what is seen here anteriorly, the brachial plexus is also in jeopardy.

Dr. Henry Khunrath Pancoast (1875-1939) has a warm place in my heart, having written his salient work while a professor at the University of Pennsylvania. I used the Pancoast Library in our department while researching for this book. Dr. Johann Friedrich Horner (1831-1886) was a Swiss ophthalmologist.

Notes

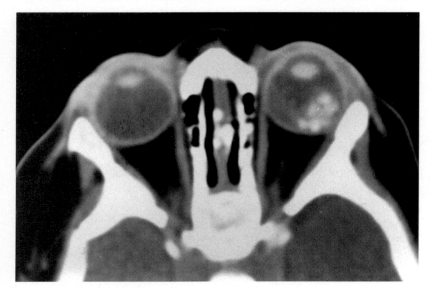

1. Where is the "third eye"? The "third testicle"?
2. How often do retinoblastomas calcify?
3. Why are retinoblastomas often bright on T1W MRI scans?
4. Why do patients with bilateral retinoblastomas develop head and neck cancers?

CASE 38

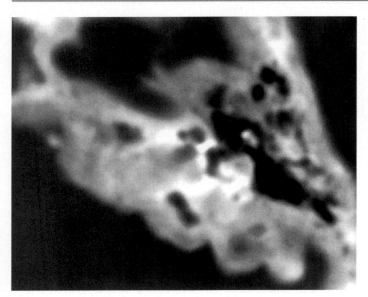

1. How can Paget's disease and fibrous dysplasia be differentiated?
2. What structures of the temporal bone are usually spared in Paget's disease?
3. What are the MRI characteristics of Paget's disease?
4. Is the skull base a common site for malignant degeneration of Paget's disease?

Retinoblastoma

1. The pineal gland (because of the coincidence of primitive neoplasms of the pineal gland and bilateral retinoblastoma, and because of the occurrence of germ cell tumors in the pineal gland) is called the third eye and the third testicle.

2. Ninety-five percent of the time.

3. It may be the calcification, retinal detachment associated with the tumor, or other paramagnetism that accounts for the high signal intensity on T1W MRI.

4. There is an oncogene that predisposes to soft tissue sarcomas in irradiated fields associated with retinoblastomas. The radiation effect may be the "second hit" in the multiple hit theory of neoplasm development.

Reference

Provenzale JM, Weber AL, Klintworth GK, McLendon RE: Radiologic-pathologic correlation: bilateral retinoblastoma with coexistent pinealoblastoma (trilateral retinoblastoma), *AJNR Am J Neuroradiol* 16:157-165, 1995.

Cross-Reference

Neuroradiology: THE REQUISITES, pp 284-286.

Comment

Retinoblastoma is a diagnosis of early childhood (90% of cases present before age 5) in which the patient presents with leukokoria. It is the most common intraocular malignancy in a child. Bilaterality occurs in about one third of patients in the sporadic cases, but at a higher rate (up to 90%) when the disease is familial (10%). Trilateral retinoblastomas refer to bilateral ocular lesions with a pineal mass (often a pineoblastoma presenting a few years after the ocular lesions) and are seen in less than 5% of cases of bilateral retinoblastomas. The differential diagnosis of a calcified ocular mass includes Coats' disease (congenital retinal telangiectasia), persistent hyperplastic primary vitreous, retinal fibroplasia, *Toxocara* infection (from canine *Toxocara* larvae), and retinal astrocytoma. Retinoblastoma occurs earlier in life than most of these other entities.

MRI may be recommended in some cases to assess for tumor spread along the optic nerve or along the optic nerve sheath and/or subarachnoid space from which the tumor may gain access to the intracranial compartment. Although there may be high signal on T1W scans, necrosis may also occur, so the signal intensity on T1W and T2W MRI may vary. The gadolinium-enhanced fat-suppressed scans are important to perform to look for optic nerve or cerebrospinal fluid (CSF) seeding.

Notes

Paget's Disease of the Temporal Bone

1. Usually they occur in two different populations—Paget's disease occurring in the elderly patient, and fibrous dysplasia occurring in the young adult. It is said that with fibrous dysplasia there is preservation of the cortex of the bone; this is not seen in Paget's disease, in which diffuse infiltration of the bone may occur. Paget's disease does not have a typical "ground glass" appearance.

2. The inner ear structures.

3. Variable signal intensity on T1W and T2W scans with heterogeneous contrast enhancement.

4. No, this is relatively rare.

Reference

Ginsberg LE, Elster AD, Moody DM: MRI of Paget disease with temporal bone involvement presenting with sensorineural hearing loss, *J Comput Assist Tomogr* 16:314-316, 1992.

Cross-Reference

Neuroradiology: THE REQUISITES, pp 352, 390, 495.

Comment

Hearing impairment with calvarial Paget's disease (reported in 30% to 50% of patients with skull involvement) may be on a sensorineural basis as a result of the expanded bone of the internal auditory canal compressing the nerves or because of involvement of the labyrinth. As can be seen in this case, the patient has nearly complete obliteration of the left internal auditory canal. Conductive hearing loss resulting from middle and external ear involvement is a rare cause of hearing loss with Paget's disease. Paget's disease goes through a lytic phase in the skull (osteoporosis circumscripta), then a mixed phase in which the osteoclasts and osteoblasts fight for territory, followed by a blastic phase. The highly vascular nature of the disease may actually cause tinnitus and/or congestive heart failure in the elderly adult. Shunting in the bone may occur. Mixed signal intensity as a result of osteolysis, hemorrhage, vascular flow channels, fat, and dense bone is present on T1W and T2W scans.

Sir James Paget (1814-1899), a British surgeon, is credited with describing this common bone disease. An adult patient who complains of having to buy larger and larger sized hats is the classic story for Paget's disease. In a child with open sutures, one worries about hydrocephalus and/or acromegaly for the same complaint.

Notes

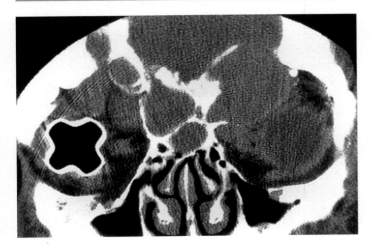
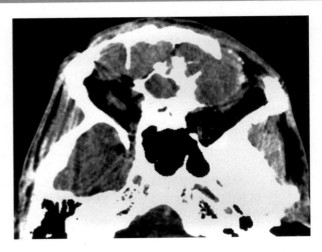
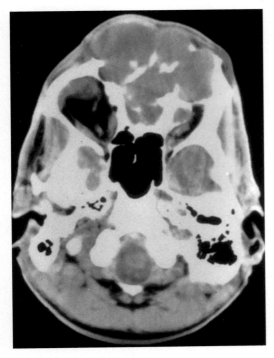

1. What is the least likely site for a mucocele?

2. Why are mucoceles often bright on T1W scans?

3. What is the sine qua non of mucoceles on CT and MRI?

4. Can cancers cause mucoceles?

Mucoceles

1. The sphenoid sinus.

2. Because of high protein.

3. On CT, the expanded sinus walls with ostium obstructed. On MRI, the peripheral rim enhancement in an expanded sinus.

4. Absolutely, if they obstruct ostia.

Reference

Lanzieri CF, Shah M, Krauss D, Lavertu P: Use of gadolinium-enhanced MR imaging for differentiating mucoceles from neoplasms in the paranasal sinuses, *Radiology* 178:425-428, 1991.

Cross-Reference

Neuroradiology: THE REQUISITES, pp 299-300.

Comment

Lanzieri's article nicely points out the value of gadolinium-enhanced scanning in differentiating mucoceles from neoplasms of the paranasal sinuses. MRI signal intensity characteristics could separate the two in 63% of the cases, but gadolinium-enhanced scans had 91.4% accuracy. Even with coexisting neoplasm and mucocele, gadolinium-enhanced MRI was nearly twice as accurate as unenhanced MRI. Go with it, it will save you—solid enhancement is tumor, rim enhancement is inflammatory. Mucoceles are most common in the frontoethmoidal region as a result of frontoethmoidal recess (nasofrontal duct) obstruction. Another setting in which mucoceles are fairly common is after frontal sinus osteoplastic flap obliteration. In this case regrowth of mucosa may produce autonomously secreting mucous glands that produce an expansile collection behind the surgically occluded ostia. With nowhere else to go, the sinus balloons out.

Patients with frontoethmoidal mucoceles usually present with headache, diplopia, and/or proptosis. The differential diagnosis includes an encephalocele, so MRI may be useful. Treatment of mucoceles may consist of relieving the site of blocked drainage. However, when dealing with multiloculated mucoceles, as in this case, one may have to try to enter each and every cell to completely relieve the process. This is still best attempted via an endoscopic approach.

Notes

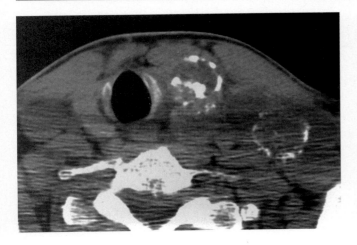
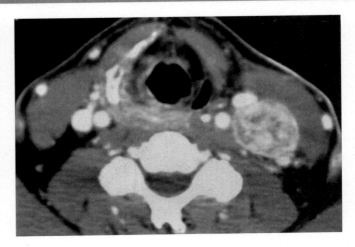
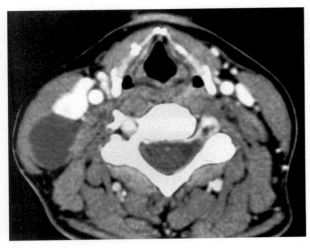

1. List the diverse appearances of thyroid carcinoma lymph node metastases.

2. How often is nodal disease the chief complaint of a patient with thyroid carcinoma?

3. What is lateral aberrant thyroid tissue?

4. What is the most common site of distant metastases from papillary thyroid cancer?

Metastatic Thyroid Carcinoma Nodes

1. Cystic nodes, vascular nodes, calcified nodes, hemorrhagic nodes, and colloid-containing nodes.

2. Approximately 50% of the time.

3. Although it used to be thought that aberrant thyroid tissue could be extrinsic to the thyroid gland in the lateral aspect of the neck, most people now believe that this represents lymph node metastases from a thyroid papillary carcinoma.

4. The lung.

Reference

Som PM, Brandwein M, Lidov M, Lawson W, Biller HF: The varied presentations of papillary thyroid carcinoma cervical nodal disease: CT and MR findings, *AJNR Am J Neuroradiol* 15:1123-1128, 1994.

Cross-Reference

Neuroradiology: THE REQUISITES, p 441.

Comment

Of all of the neoplasms to produce lymphadenopathy, papillary carcinoma of the thyroid gland produces the wildest appearances. Cystic, calcified, hypervascular, proteinaceous, or bloody nodes can be seen anywhere in the head and neck. Therefore the nodes may be dense or low attenuation on CT. Calcifications in the nodes may be rim or speckly; enhancement may be rim, solid, or nonexistent; hemorrhage may or may not be present. On MRI the signal intensity is also variable with high or low T1W intensity. Nodes may be anywhere—retropharyngeal, intraparotid, periesophageal, paratracheal, jugular chain, mediastinal, and delphian (pretracheal). The nodes may be tiny or massive. Iodine-131 imaging after thyroidectomy may be the best way to visualize all of the metastatic adenopathy of a thyroid malignancy. Around 60% of papillary and 50% of follicular thyroid cancers show avid iodine uptake.

The mortality rate from thyroid cancer increases nearly fifteenfold once a thyroid carcinoma escapes the thyroid capsule (2.5% versus 40%). Local or regional disease leads to death more commonly than do distant metastases. Nonetheless, a thyroid primary tumor should be suspected with a "miliary pattern" of nodules on a chest x-ray, with a bubbly lytic bone lesion, with hypervascular metastases anywhere in the body, and when cervical lymphadenopathy is present but the primary tumor is occult.

Notes

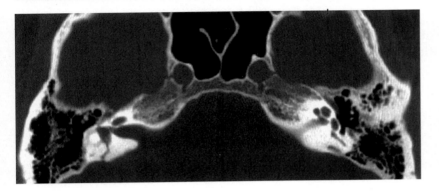
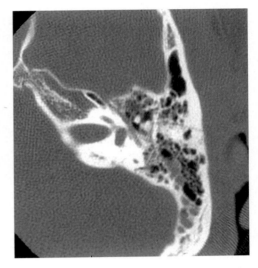

1. Which are more likely to disrupt the facial nerve, longitudinal (horizontal) or transverse (vertical) fractures of the temporal bone?

2. Which are more likely to cause ossicular disruption, longitudinal or transverse fractures of the temporal bone?

3. What is the most common orientation of a temporal bone fracture?

4. What is the most common site of a transverse fracture of the temporal bone?

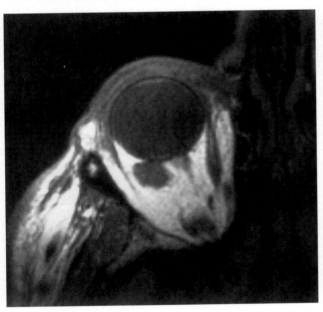
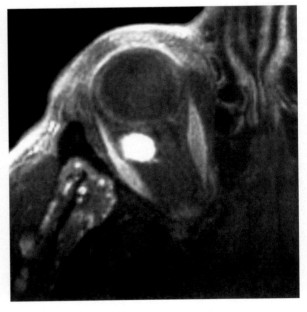

1. What is the most common intraconal tumor in the adult?

2. What does the differential diagnosis of a highly enhancing mass in the orbit include?

3. Are calcification and phleboliths commonly seen in hemangiomas in this location?

4. What is the age range of patients with capillary hemangiomas of the orbit?

CASE 41

Transverse Fracture (Figure on Left) and Longitudinal Fracture with Ossicular Dislocation (Figure on Right) of the Right Temporal Bone

1. Transverse fractures.

2. Longitudinal fractures.

3. Trick question—oblique fracture (combination of transverse and longitudinal fractures).

4. Either through the midportion of the temporal bone, so that the fracture traverses the distal labyrinthine segment or geniculate ganglion of the facial nerve, or through the vestibule (as shown here).

Reference

Backous DD, Minor LB, Niparko JK: Trauma to the external auditory canal and temporal bone, *Otolaryngol Clin North Am* 29:853-866, 1996.

Cross-Reference

Neuroradiology: THE REQUISITES, p 355.

Comment

Eighty percent of temporal bone fractures have a predominantly longitudinal orientation (though most really are obliquely oriented). Disruption through the roof of the temporal bone is more common with transverse fractures, but tympanic membrane rupture, external auditory canal fractures, incudostapedial dislocation, and conductive hearing loss are more common with longitudinal fractures. Transverse fractures usually cross the bony labyrinth and have a higher rate of vestibular symptoms than do longitudinal fractures. Oblique fractures tend to have clinical characteristics similar to those of longitudinal fractures. Despite the fact that transverse fractures affect the facial nerve more frequently, because longitudinally oriented fractures are so much more common than transversely oriented ones, longitudinal fractures account for more instances of facial nerve injury than do transverse fractures. It's a numbers game really.

Any patient with head trauma and air-fluid levels or opacification of the middle ear or mastoid air cells should probably have a dedicated (1-mm thick sections) study of the temporal bones to look for fractures. Often, because the patient is neurologically compromised, there is a delay in recognizing the temporal bone injury. The traumatologists may be screaming at the patient and saying he or she is unresponsive or searching for the central source of a facial nerve injury, when in fact the problem lies in conductive or sensorineural hearing loss or transection of the facial nerve caused by the temporal bone fracture. The temporal bone fracture may also be a source of intracranial air and/or subsequent meningitis.

Notes

CASE 42

Orbital Hemangioma

1. A cavernous hemangioma.

2. Hemangiomas, varices of the superior ophthalmic vein, aneurysms, fistulae, hypervascular metastases, normal enlarged veins, and hemangiopericytomas.

3. No.

4. Under 3 years of age.

Reference

Wilms G, Raat H, Dom R, Thywissen C, Demaerel P, Dralands G, Baert AL: Orbital cavernous hemangioma: findings on sequential Gd-enhanced MRI, *J Comput Assist Tomogr* 19: 548-551, 1995.

Cross-Reference

Neuroradiology: THE REQUISITES, pp 296-298.

Comment

Orbital hemangiomas are well-circumscribed encapsulated masses that usually appear intraconally in the orbit. They are usually of the cavernous type and, as such, may rarely have phleboliths associated with them. The typical patient is a 40ish-year-old woman complaining of exophthalmos and orbital discomfort with diminished visual acuity. The differential diagnosis in the orbit includes a neurogenic tumor, an orbital varix, a myxoma, a lymphangioma, or a hemangiopericytoma. Pooling of contrast agents into the dilated vascular channels of the mass is characteristic on dynamic scanning, similar to what has been described with hemangiomas of the liver. Distinguishing this lesion from a varix may necessitate vascular imaging (MRA, CTA) because a varix does not have soft tissue associated with it. A Valsalva's maneuver or coronal supine head down imaging often demonstrates marked enlargement of a varix over its baseline size, but there may also be some increase in volume with some hemangiomas. One would not expect to see size changes with schwannomas, myxomas, or other solitary masses in the orbit such as lymphoma or pseudotumor.

Cavernous hemangiomas of the orbit are compressible lesions consisting of large vascular channels. As such, one of the distinguishing features of these entities is that they do not displace or remodel orbital structures in their course. Therefore by the time they present clinically they are larger in size than other lesions. They may also be found incidentally. Thrombosis of the vascular channels of the lesions may lead to acute symptoms.

Notes

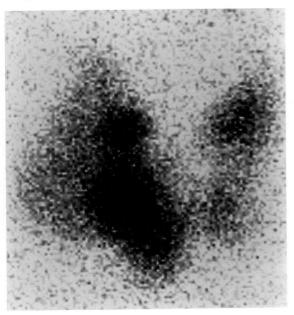

1. Is the risk of cancer in a cold expanding nodule higher or lower in a goiter than in a normal thyroid gland?
2. What are the two most common causes of thyroid goiter worldwide?
3. What is the most common cause of hypothyroidism in the United States?
4. What is the most common cause of hyperthyroidism in the United States?

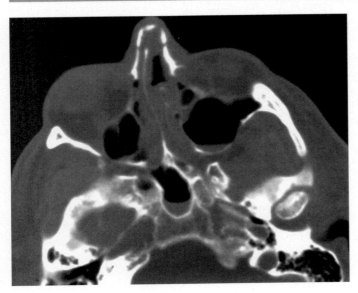

1. What is the sine qua non of acute sinusitis?
2. What role do plain films have in the evaluation of patients before surgical management of chronic sinusitis?
3. What are the major structures of the ostiomeatal complex?
4. What is the significance of a concha bullosa?

CASE 43

Goiter

1. It is very, very close; perhaps a little less in a goiter.

2. Iodine deficiency and Hashimoto's thyroiditis.

3. Hashimoto's thyroiditis and glandular obliteration for hyperthyroidism run "neck and neck" for number one.

4. Graves' disease.

Reference
Hurley DL, Gharib H: Evaluation and management of multinodular goiter, *Otolaryngol Clin North Am* 29:527-540, 1996.

Cross-Reference
Neuroradiology: THE REQUISITES, pp 438-439.

Comment
A goiter is a big thyroid gland. The terms nontoxic goiter and toxic goiter refer to the hormonal state of the gland, with the latter often used synonymously with Graves' disease. A goiter may have one or more nodules in it, and goiters are more common in women and in the elderly. Most goiters are discovered as asymptomatic masses during routine physical examination. A fixed, growing, or hard nodule is suspicious for malignancy, and the presence of vocal cord paralysis, superior vena cava syndrome, Horner's syndrome, or adenopathy should increase the suspicion of neoplasm even if the nodule occurs within a multinodular goiter. Surgical intervention is warranted with symptom-producing tracheal narrowing (over 50%), for cosmesis, for suspicion of concomitant malignancy and for persistent hyperthyroidism (nodular toxic goiter). In patients in whom Hashimoto's thyroiditis is a cause of the goiter, one must worry about the propensity for lymphoma.

Goiters have heterogeneous appearances on all modalities: (1) echogenic and echopenic areas on ultrasound; (2) hot, cold, and/or warm areas on scintigraphy; (3) dense or lucent areas on CT; and (4) mixed intensity zones on MRI. Because goiters may undergo hemorrhage or colloidal degradation, they may show areas of hyperdensity on CT and hyperintensity on T1W MRI.

Notes

CASE 44

Acute Sinusitis (Not a Trauma Case)

1. Air-fluid levels.

2. None.

3. The maxillary sinus ostium, infundibulum, uncinate process, middle meatus, anterior ethmoid air cells (bulla), hiatus semilunaris, and middle turbinate.

4. Its presence means little—it's the size that counts; that is, does it obstruct?

Reference
Yousem DM: Imaging of sinonasal inflammatory disease: state of the art, *Radiology* 188:303-314, 1993.

Cross-Reference
Neuroradiology: THE REQUISITES, pp 363-368.

Comment
The work-up of a patient with chronic sinusitis has changed over recent years because of the advent of experienced intranasal endoscopists. Acute bouts of sinusitis are typically treated medically, and the diagnosis is usually made on clinical grounds. Imaging is usually not required at all unless confusion about the diagnosis is present. Patients with recurrent or intractable sinusitis may be referred to an otorhinolaryngologist for evaluation. Most patients who have recurrent or chronic symptoms (debilitating headache, facial pain, or congestion) despite medical therapy undergo office intranasal endoscopy. Based on the endoscopic findings and the clinical symptomatology, the patient may be treated with additional courses of long-term antibiotics, steroids, intranasal mucolytics, antiinflammatory drugs, and/or decongestants. If the patient fails to respond to intensive medical therapy and the initial endoscopic findings suggest surgically correctable abnormalities, imaging may be requested preoperatively.

To eliminate the effects of reversible sinus congestion, patients undergoing CT for evaluation of chronic sinus disease are best scanned 4 to 6 weeks after maximal medical therapy, and not during an acute infection. Some radiology departments administer nasal spray decongestants or antihistaminics to reduce reversible mucosal edema before putting the patient in the scanner. This aids in assessing the nonreversible sinus disease. Coronal CT scans that mimic the view of the endoscopist are evaluated for anatomy and normal variants of which the surgeon must be aware to plan effective functional endoscopic sinus surgery. One must be wary of areas of dehiscence along the cribriform plate, lamina papyracea, optic nerves, and carotid arteries.

Notes

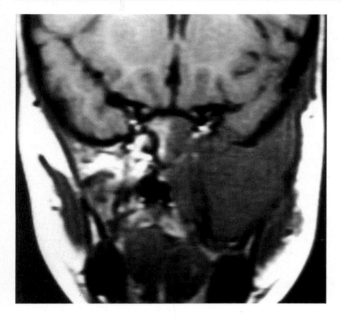

1. What is the significance of parameningeal rhabdomyosarcomas?

2. What is the incidence of hemorrhage in rhabdomyosarcomas?

3. What is the difference between the lateral pterygoid muscle and the medial pterygoid muscle, temporalis muscle, and masseter muscle?

4. What are the most common locations of rhabdomyosarcomas of the head and neck?

CASE 46

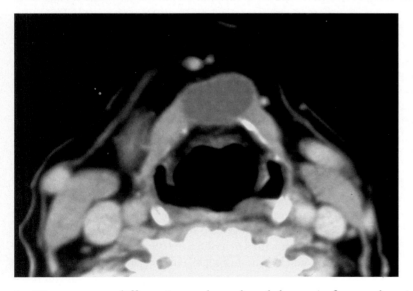

1. How can one differentiate a thyroglossal duct cyst from a thymic cyst?

2. In which does cancer occur more frequently, a thyroglossal duct cyst or ectopic lingual thyroid gland tissue?

3. What percentage of congenital cystic lesions of the neck are thyroglossal duct cysts?

4. What percentage of thyroglossal duct cysts occur at the suprahyoid, hyoid, and infrahyoid levels?

CASE 45

Masticator Space Rhabdomyosarcoma

1. They have a much worse prognosis than nonparameningeal rhabdomyosarcomas.

2. Approximately 30%.

3. It is the only muscle of mastication that opens the jaw.

4. The orbit, temporal bone, and masticator space.

Reference

Odell PF: Head and neck sarcomas: a review, *J Otolaryngol* 25:7-13, 1996.

Cross-Reference

Neuroradiology: THE REQUISITES, pp 424-429, 435.

Comment

This is a child, and this lesion crawls up the suprazygomatic portion of the left masticator space along the temporalis muscle—put the two together and you have a rhabdomyosarcoma. Invasion into foramen ovale is present, and there is tumor in the middle cranial fossa.

Rhabdomyosarcomas represent 50% of all soft tissue sarcomas in children, and sarcomas account for 6% of all pediatric cancers. Rhabdomyosarcomas of the head and neck are usually of the less aggressive embryonal variety. Staging takes place after surgical resection and is graded from 1 to 4: (1) localized complete resection, (2) presumed microscopic residua, (3) gross residua, and (4) distant metastases. This staging system is now controversial because many centers advocate radiation and chemotherapy over surgical treatment. Chemotherapy (often prolonged over years) has led to dramatic improvements in the prognosis of head and neck rhabdomyosarcomas over the past decade, such that combined radiation therapy and chemotherapy compete with surgical treatment for the best cure rate. Typical 5-year survival rates are 60%. Orbital rhabdomyosarcomas have the best prognosis; parameningeal ones with meningeal infiltration have the worst. Adult onset and alveolar type histology are associated with a worse prognosis. Other soft tissue tumors of the masticator space to be considered include synovial sarcomas (cystic, calcified, hemorrhagic), minor salivary gland tumors (homogeneous), neurogenic tumors (along neuronal pathways), hemangio(pericyto)mas (markedly enhancing), and lymphomas (bland with systemic symptoms associated).

Notes

CASE 46

Thyroglossal Duct Cyst

1. Thyroglossal duct cysts occur along the tract of the thyroglossal duct, usually infrahyoid in location and usually in the midline. They may be embedded in the strap muscles in front of the hyoid bone or larynx, a finding that is pathognomonic for thyroglossal duct cysts. A thymic cyst descends into the mediastinum via the left and right thymopharyngeal ducts, remnants of the third branchial pouch. A thymic cyst may be associated with the thyroid gland but is usually off midline and more commonly below the thyroid gland, unlike a thyroglossal duct cyst.

2. Lingual thyroid gland tissue.

3. Approximately 90%.

4. Twenty-five percent occur suprahyoid, 15% hyoid, and 60% infrahyoid.

Reference

Wadsworth DT, Siegel MJ: Thyroglossal duct cysts: variability of sonographic findings, *AJR Am J Roentgenol* 163:1475-1477, 1994.

Cross-Reference

Neuroradiology: THE REQUISITES, pp 438, 444.

Comment

Thyroglossal duct cysts are the most common congenital cysts in the neck, and they have been discovered with increasing frequency thanks to cross-sectional imaging techniques. As a result, there has been a shift in the reporting of the lesions, with most presenting as incidental asymptomatic masses. This is the "Tornwaldt cyst" of the lower neck. Whereas the thyroid gland in the neck may be absent in up to 70% of cases of lingual thyroid glands, it is usually present and normally functioning in patients with thyroglossal duct cysts. Migration of the thyroid from the foramen cecum of the tongue to the lower neck occurs during the third to seventh weeks of embryonic development. It is very rare (approximately 1% of cases) for a carcinoma to develop in a thyroglossal duct cyst—when it occurs, it is usually a papillary carcinoma (86% of cases). Twenty-five percent of thyroglossal duct cysts are off midline. The majority are hypoechoic (not anechoic) on ultrasound, presumably because of infection, hemorrhage, or high protein content. Dermoids, in the differential diagnosis of a midline neck lesion, are echogenic on ultrasound and are usually seen anterior to the strap muscles.

In the Sistrunk procedure, the cyst and a portion of the hyoid bone and base of the tongue may be removed in an attempt to completely eradicate any remnants of the duct. This prevents recurrence.

Notes

CASE 47

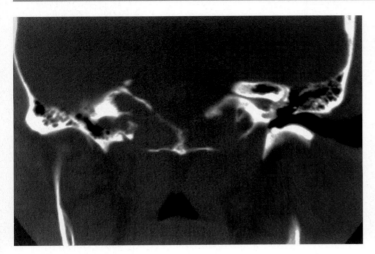 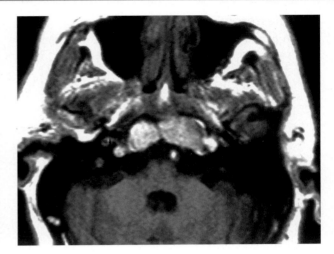

1. What does the differential diagnosis of a cholesterol granuloma of the petrous apex include?

2. What is the danger in not treating a cholesterol granuloma of the petrous apex?

3. What should one consider with a calcified lesion at the petrous apex?

4. In what percentage of patients is the petrous apex aerated?

CASE 48

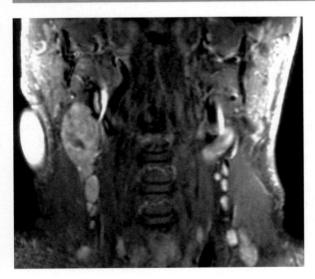

1. What does the differential diagnosis of large lymph nodes and enlarged Waldeyer's ring tissue include?

2. What does the differential diagnosis of large lymph nodes and a skin lesion include?

3. What does the differential diagnosis of large lymph nodes and enlarged nodular salivary glands include?

4. What does the differential diagnosis of large lymph nodes with calcification include?

Cholesterol Granuloma

1. A petrous apex mucocele and an epidermoid tumor because both can have high signal intensity on T1W scans.

2. Complications of cholesterol granulomas include pseudo-aneurysms of the petrous carotid artery, chemical meningitis, and septic thrombophlebitis.

3. A calcified giant aneurysm of the petrous carotid artery, chordoma, chondrosarcoma, and meningioma of the petrous apex.

4. Approximately 30% to 40%.

Reference

Isaacson JE, Sismanis A: Cholesterol granuloma cyst of the petrous apex, *Ear Nose Throat J* 75:425-429, 1996.

Cross-Reference

Neuroradiology: THE REQUISITES, pp 330, 353.

Comment

Cholesterol granulomas (also known as blue dome cysts, chocolate cysts, cholesterol cysts, giant cholesterol cysts) are characteristically bright on T1W scans and are more dense than epidermoids on CT. Cholesterol granulomas are the most common primary expansile lesion of the petrous apex. At my institution, cholesterol granuloma drainage may be achieved endoscopically by placement of drainage catheters from the sphenoid sinus into the petrous apex. This possibility for treatment depends on the proximity of those two structures to each other and the degree of aeration of the two. This is not definitive surgery, but because of the nearness of cholesterol granulomas to the carotid arteries, Meckel's cave (the fifth cranial nerve), the sixth cranial nerve, and the petrosal sinuses, most patients opt for the least invasive surgery that relieves symptoms. The alternative is skull base/neurosurgery.

Congenital cholesteatomas are better termed epidermoids of the temporal bone to distinguish them from acquired cholesteatomas. In the temporal bones epidermoids may occur in the middle ear, near the geniculate ganglion, and at the petrous apex—cholesterol granulomas are usually confined to the petrous apex or postoperative cavities. Epidermoids are due to congenital epithelial rests, and the temporal bone is the most common site in the calvaria in which they occur. Calvarial epidermoids are of low density with well-defined borders on CT; low intensity is *usually* seen on T1W scans. *Rarely* they are bright on T1W scans. Treatment for these two entities is different. Epidermoids require complete removal, whereas cholesterol granulomas (and petrous apex mucoceles, the third player in the region) are usually treated with marsupialization for drainage.

Notes

Multiple Lymph Nodes Secondary to Squamous Cell Carcinoma

1. Lymphoma, mononucleosis, HIV positivity, and AIDS.

2. Kaposi's sarcoma, sarcoidosis (erythema multiforme), lymphoma, Kikuchi's disease, cancer, cat-scratch fever, mycobacterial infection, and actinomycosis.

3. HIV positivity, AIDS, Sjögren's syndrome, sarcoidosis, cat-scratch fever, Kimura's disease, and lymphoma.

4. Thyroid carcinoma, treated lymphoma, silicosis, sarcoidosis, and tuberculosis.

Reference

van den Brekel MWM, Castelijns JA, Snow GB: Imaging of cervical lymphadenopathy, *Neuroimaging Clin N Am* 6: 417-434, 1996.

Cross-Reference

Neuroradiology: THE REQUISITES, pp 380, 403-408.

Comment

Staging of lymph nodes depends on size [no nodes (N0), <3 cm (N1), >3 cm but <6 cm (N2), >6 cm (N3)], multiplicity (N2b), and laterality (N2c). Palpation of lymph nodes has false positive and negative rates between 20% and 40%, so imaging can be useful to accurately stage the extent of disease for squamous cell carcinoma. Microscopic disease may occur in over 20% of patients with N0 necks depending on site of origin. The bases of the tongue, pharynx, and supraglottic larynx have sufficiently high rates of occult metastases to warrant elective treatment. According to van den Brekel, measuring the short axis of a node on axial scanning and using 9 mm (up to 11 mm for jugulodigastric nodes) as the minimum cutoff yields the best combination of sensitivity (70%) and specificity (86%) for all nodes in the neck of a patient with squamous cell carcinoma. For patients who have N0 necks, one would have to use a smaller size (approximately 6 mm) to achieve reasonable sensitivity (78%), but at a cost of specificity (58%). Ultrasound-guided fine needle aspiration appears to be the most accurate means for staging lymph nodes of the neck—the technique is rarely used in American practice and is time and cost intensive to perform.

When looking at nodes, the presence of extranodal spread—that is, outside the node's capsule—is very important because the long-term prognosis is much worse once extranodal spread is present. Add in fixation to a vital structure like the carotid artery, prevertebral muscles, or vertebral body, and the long-term prognosis is dismal. Twenty-three percent of nodes less than or equal to 1 cm in size have extracapsular extension, the presence of which decreases 5-year survival by 50%. The presence of lymphadenopathy cuts the 5-year prognosis in half, and bilaterality of adenopathy is also a poor prognostic sign.

Notes

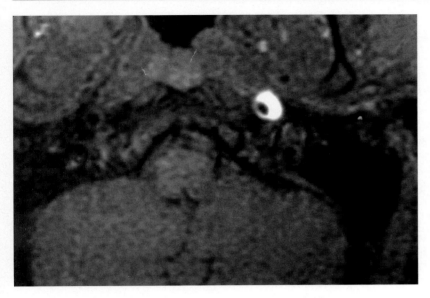

1. What are the likely symptoms in a patient with this entity?

2. What are the benefits of fat-suppressed T1W scans?

3. What disease entities are predisposed to carotid dissection?

4. What are the complications of carotid dissection?

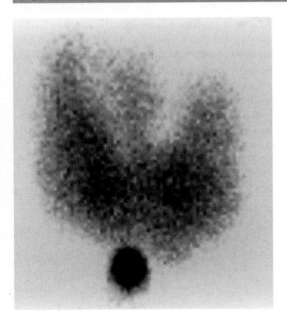

1. What are the serologic markers for Graves' disease?

2. How often do patients with Graves' disease develop thyroid ophthalmopathy?

3. What is the rate of malignancy for a nodule that is hot on technetium Tc 99m pertechnetate scanning, but cold on iodine-123 (discordant nodules)?

4. Is the rate of malignancy in a patient with multiple cold nodules the same as that in a patient with solitary nodules?

Internal Carotid Artery Dissection

1. Neck pain, neurologic deficit (stroke), Horner's syndrome, and/or transient ischemia attacks.

2. With fat suppression, one knows that the high signal intensity around the blood vessel is most likely to represent blood products as opposed to perivascular fat.

3. Fibromuscular dysplasia, cystic medial necrosis, Marfan syndrome, severe cervical head trauma, chiropractic manipulations, homocystinuria, Ehlers-Danlos syndrome, and hypocoagulable states.

4. Pseudoaneurysm formation, occlusion, and stroke.

Reference
Ozdoba C, Sturzenegger M, Schroth G: Internal carotid artery dissection: MR imaging features and clinical-radiologic correlation, *Radiology* 199:191-198, 1996.

Cross-Reference
Neuroradiology: THE REQUISITES, pp 55-57, 409-410.

Comment
MRI with MRA is probably the best study to use to look for internal carotid artery dissection. It is particularly elegant when fat suppression has been applied, which allows the wall hematoma to be visualized opposite a dark (suppressed) background on unenhanced T1W scans. The MRA is icing on the cake. There are areas where the MRI is fraught with problems—any time the vessel begins to turn in plane (seen with the vertebral arteries at C1-C2 and the petrous carotid), as a result of flow-related enhancement, or if there is huge atherosclerotic plaque with intraplaque hemorrhage. Most of the time, however, the MRI does the job. On the MRA, it behooves the radiologist to look at the source images and include a phase contrast MRA (in which the high intensity wall hematoma is nulled, unlike the time of flight MRA) if confusion exists. Following these patients with MRI and MRA to determine the development of pseudoaneurysms is warranted because carotid "blow-out" or thromboembolism from the aneurysm can be catastrophic. Most clinicians will anticoagulate with aspirin as treatment for dissections.

Lately, endovascular treatment of cervical carotid artery dissections with or without pseudoaneurysms has gained favor. Stents to keep the carotid artery open or the pseudoaneurysm out can be used but are usually reserved for those individuals who are throwing emboli into the intracranial circulation or who have an enlarging pseudoaneurysm. Stents may also be the wave of the future for atherosclerosis of the cervical carotid artery—you heard it here first!

Notes

Graves' Disease on Thyroid Scan

1. Antibodies to the TSH receptor, thyroperoxidase, thyroglobulin–antithyroid microsomal antibodies, thyroid stimulating antibody.

2. One third of the time.

3. Less than 3%.

4. No, the rate is slightly greater (4.7% versus 4.1%) in a patient with solitary nodules.

Reference
Prummel MF, Wiersinga WM: Smoking and risk of Graves' disease, *JAMA* 269:479-482, 1993.

Cross-Reference
Neuroradiology: THE REQUISITES, p 439.

Comment
Although Graves' disease (from Robert James Graves, an Irish physician, 1796-1853) is considered an autoimmune disorder, there does seem to be some link to smoking, especially in those patients who develop Graves' ophthalmopathy. Smoking may affect T cells, which in turn may prevent the immunologic attack on thyroid antigens that causes Graves' disease. In fact, the severity of Graves' ophthalmopathy appears to correlate with amount of cigarettes smoked.

In patients who are hyperthyroid, Graves' disease is far and away the most common cause. However, one should also consider a solitary toxic adenoma, the hypermetabolic phase of thyroiditis, multinodular toxic goiter, exogenous thyroid hormone abuse or overdosage, and ectopic sources of thyroid hormone (struma ovarii, struma cardii). The scintigraphic uptake of the tracer is not "hot" with exogenous hormone abuse and in some forms of thyroiditis, so there may be a discordance of thyroid "function" and radiotracer uptake.

Thyroid function tests (TFTs) and the 24-hour radioactive iodine uptake (RAIU) need not be concordant and may help in the differential diagnosis of thyroid pathology. If both are elevated, the differential diagnosis is Graves' disease or Marine-Lenhart disease. If the TFTs are elevated but the RAIU is normal, one should consider Plummer's disease (hyperthyroidism caused by a solitary autonomous hot nodule that suppresses the remainder of the gland), unusual forms of Graves' disease, or laboratory error. If TFTs are elevated but RAIU is depressed, the possibilities include subacute granulomatous thyroiditis, subacute lymphocytic thyroiditis, postpartum thyroiditis, and struma ovarii.

One should note the enlarged midline pyramidal lobe in this patient with Graves' disease.

Notes

Fair Game

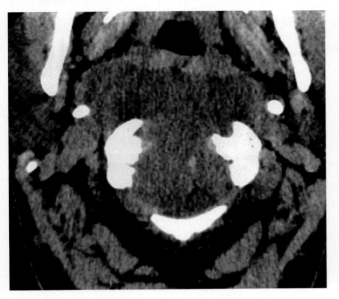
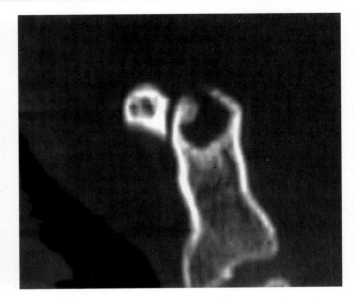

1. What structure's displacement is critical to determining that this lesion is from the skull base/posterolateral (perivertebral) space rather than the retropharyngeal space?

2. In an adult, what are the most likely causes of this mass?

3. In a child or young adult, what are the most likely diagnoses?

4. How does one distinguish between chordomas and chondrosarcomas?

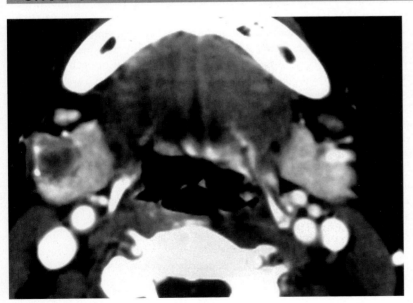

1. What is the most common tumor of the submandibular gland?

2. Are malignant tumors of the submandibular gland more common than benign tumors of the submandibular gland?

3. What are the MRI signal intensity characteristics of pleomorphic adenomas?

4. What malignancies of the salivary glands may be bright on T2W scans?

Chordoma

1. The longus muscles that are displaced anteriorly by the mass, identifying it as a perivertebral space lesion.

2. Metastatic disease to bone, plasmacytoma/multiple myeloma, chordoma, chondrosarcoma, and lymphoma.

3. Chordoma, sarcoma (Ewing's, osteosarcoma), neuroblastoma, lymphoma.

4. No good criteria exist. If the lesion is more lateral, has classic chondroid matrix with whorls of calcification, or arose from a predisposing bone lesion, one should favor chondrosarcoma.

Reference

Meyers SP, Hirsch WJ Jr, Curtin HD, Barnes L, Sekhar LN, Sen C: Chordomas of the skull base: MR features, *AJNR Am J Neuroradiol* 13:1627-1636, 1992.

Cross-Reference

Neuroradiology: THE REQUISITES, pp 436-437.

Comment

The distinction between chordomas and chondrosarcomas has elicited a couple of hundred articles in the radiology literature with few if any definitive findings used to separate the two. This is also reflected in the neuropathologic literature, in which chondroid chordomas exist as a category of chondrosarcomas. In my experience, chordomas, which often appear gelatinous at surgery, tend to be brighter on T2W and fluid attenuation inversion recovery (FLAIR) images than chondrosarcomas, which are a little more cellular. Calcified matrix, irregular margins, paramedian location, and foci of heterogeneous density and signal intensity may be seen with both entities. If the lesion classically is centered on the petrooccipital synchondrosis, one should favor a chondrosarcoma. The head and neck is the primary site in only 6.7% of all chondrosarcomas. They classically are heterogeneous on T2W scans and enhance avidly.

A few fun facts about chordomas: They occur in the upper cervical spine and sacrococcygeal region in addition to the clivus. They have the characteristic physaliferous (bubbly/vacuolated) cells. Nonneoplastic remnants of the notochord called ecchordoses occur along the clivus in 2% of autopsied patients. Headaches and a sixth nerve palsy are the most common presentations of chordomas.

Notes

Monomorphic Adenoma of the Submandibular Gland

1. Pleomorphic adenoma (benign mixed tumor).

2. No, benign tumors are ever so slightly more common than malignant tumors of the submandibular gland.

3. They are usually isointense to muscle on T1W scans and very bright on T2W scans. They enhance avidly.

4. Low grade mucoepidermoid carcinomas, adenoid cystic carcinomas, and rarely adenocarcinomas.

Reference

Weber RS, Byers RM, Petit B, Wolf P, Ang K, Luna M: Submandibular gland tumors: adverse histologic factors and therapeutic implications, *Arch Otolaryngol Head Neck Surg* 116:1055-1060, 1990.

Cross-Reference

Neuroradiology: THE REQUISITES, pp 385-386, 415, 419-420, 424.

Comment

Monomorphic adenomas of the salivary glands include myoepitheliomas, oncocytic adenomas, and canalicular adenomas. These tumors are much less common than pleomorphic adenomas at all sites. Both types of lesions most often present in the submandibular region as a painless lump felt by the patient, and the clinician tries to distinguish the lesion from an adjacent lymph node. The radiologist can help in this regard. Furthermore, with a lesion that has well-defined margins, is bright on T2W scans, and is uniformly enhancing, you should suggest a benign tumor. If there is any possibility that the lesion may be related to calculus disease (i.e., a Kuttner tumor), one should recommend CT because calculi may be missed on MRI. Sialography has no role.

The absence of inflammatory stranding in the subcutaneous fat is the best indication that this lesion is not an abscess. The eccentric nature of the mass also suggests a neoplasm over an abscess. The bright areas on the periphery are vessels, not calculi—another reason to perform pre- and postcontrast scans for lesions of the salivary glands. The confusing features of this lesion are the absence of well-defined margins and its irregular contour because elsewhere in the body these findings may suggest a malignancy. Salivary gland neoplasms do not follow the rules in this regard—regular margins may be found with malignancies, and ill-defined margins are not incompatible with benign tumors.

Notes

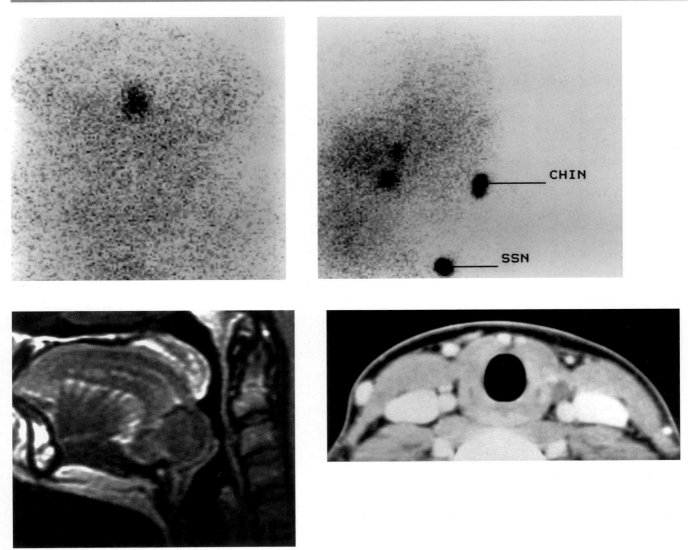

1. What is the most important finding on these figures?
2. Is the incidence of cancer higher or lower in a lingual thyroid gland than in normally located thyroid tissue?
3. How does a lingual thyroid gland appear on CT?
4. Why do these lesions often present in adolescence?

Lingual Thyroid Gland*

1. No thyroid tissue in the neck.

2. The same.

3. Very dense before and after contrast enhancement.

4. As TSH levels increase in adolescence, the tissue hypertrophies and causes symptoms.

Reference

Williams JD, Sclafani AP, Slupchinskij O, Douge C: Evaluation and management of the lingual thyroid gland, *Ann Otol Rhinol Laryngol* 105:312-316, 1996.

Cross-Reference

Neuroradiology: THE REQUISITES, pp 385, 438-441.

Comment

The incidence of lingual thyroid glands in healthy individuals is only about 1 in 100,000, and they occur 4 times more often in women. Symptoms such as dysphagia, airway obstruction, and globus sensation may herald a lingual thyroid gland, which is usually located between the foramen cecum of the tongue and the epiglottis in the midline suprahyoid neck. Hemorrhage may occur into the mass, causing acute airway compromise that is particularly dangerous in the small neonatal airway. Scintigraphy is the best study to evaluate the abnormal tissue and to look for other sites of thyroid function—this obviates the need for biopsy and the subsequent risk of hemorrhage. By having the tissue suppressed with thyroid hormone, most patients can achieve relief of their symptoms as the "mass" goes down in size. During stress, adolescence, and pregnancy the mass should be monitored for precipitous enlargement.

Other sites for ectopic functioning thyroid tissue include the pericardial region, ovarian teratomas, the trachea, lateral to the jugular veins, and metastatic thyroid carcinoma. Iodine-131 scanning is probably the best way to evaluate the whole body for functioning thyroid tissue.

Notes

---

* Figures for Case 53 courtesy Sydney Heyman, MD, and Suresh Mukherji, MD.

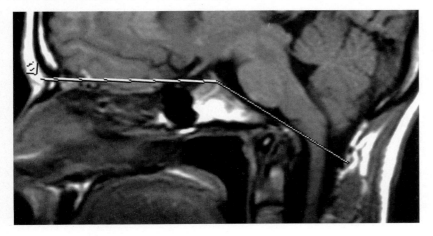

1. Define the basal angle.

2. What is the normal value for the basal angle?

3. What are the common causes of platybasia?

4. Distinguish platybasia from basilar invagination.

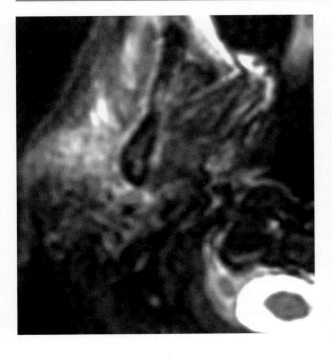 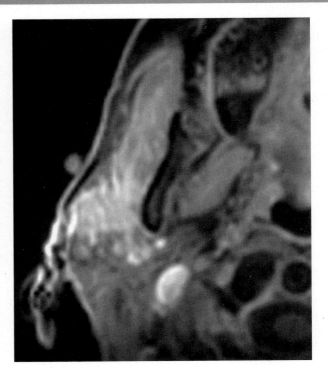

1. What is the most common cause of parotitis?

2. What is the clinical sine qua non of parotitis?

3. How can one distinguish a parotid abscess from a neoplasm?

4. Of bacterial causes of parotitis, which are most common?

Platybasia

1. Draw a line from the nasion to the tuberculum sellae and from the tuberculum sellae down the plane of the clivus to the anterior margin of the foramen magnum. This is the basal (Weneke's) angle.

2. Less than or equal to 143 degrees.

3. Cranial settling caused by Paget's disease, osteomalacia, renal osteodystrophy, Down syndrome, achondroplasia, and osteogenesis imperfecta.

4. Platybasia refers to flattening of the basal angle, whereas basal invagination reflects superior extension of the odontoid process through the plane of the hard palate and foramen magnum.

Reference

Crockard HA, Stevens JM: Craniovertebral junction anomalies in inherited disorders: part of the syndrome or caused by the disorder? *Eur J Pediatr* 154:504-512, 1995.

Cross-Reference

Neuroradiology: THE REQUISITES, p 264.

Comment

Weneke's angle is used to define platybasia. Chamberlain's line (from hard palate to posterior margin of the foramen magnum) and McGregor's lines (from hard palate to undersurface of the occiput) are used to define basilar invagination. If the dens lies greater than or equal to 5 to 7 mm above these two lines, there is basilar invagination. Basilar invagination is more common than platybasia, and Chiari I malformations may occur with either entity. Depending on the severity of the disorder (usually based on spinal cord compression), operative decompression may be required. This is particularly true if atlantoaxial dislocation coexists, as with patients who have Down syndrome, Morquio's syndrome, and other congenital disorders.

The concurrence of basilar invagination, platybasia, and a Chiari I (seen in this patient) suggests that skull base development is linked with the rhombencephalon. Compression of the brain stem or cervical cord may lead to cranial nerve symptoms, gait complaints, myelopathy, or pain syndromes. Rarely ischemia of the vertebrobasilar system may be the presenting finding, usually with the more severe cases. Surgical decompression is reserved for the more severe degrees of basilar invagination and platybasia.

Notes

Parotitis

1. Mumps (viral parotitis) paramyxovirus.

2. Purulent material able to be expressed from Stensen's duct.

3. With difficulty. Sometimes parotid abscesses lead to diffuse parotid enhancement, and the typical features of rim enhancement around a parotid abscess are not evident.

4. *Streptococcus* and *Staphylococcus* organisms.

Reference

Tunkel DE: Atypical mycobacterial adenitis presenting as a parotid abscess, *Am J Otolaryngol* 16:428-432, 1995.

Cross-Reference

Neuroradiology: THE REQUISITES, pp 175, 415.

Comment

The parotid gland may appear inflamed with many causes of cervical adenitis because there is drainage to intraparotid lymph nodes and hence sialadenitis. Nontuberculous mycobacterial parotitis probably affects the gland via nodal spread. Cytology is notoriously inaccurate in the parotid gland for distinguishing neoplasms from inflammatory lesions, and this "mass" was initially read as showing carcinoma.

Parotitis is often a quandary for the clinicians. Apparently parotid inflammation is often misinterpreted as neoplastic on parotid cytology, and by the same token, parotid neoplasms often induce an inflammatory reaction. Furthermore, any surgery on the parotid gland is complicated by the presence of the facial nerve coursing through the gland—in an inflamed gland the nerve is very hard to dissect cleanly without a greater risk of injury and subsequent paralysis. In my experience, three of the four cases in which cytology was incorrect (among 113 CT-guided aspirations I have performed) occurred with parotid lesions that were mistakenly called inflammatory or neoplastic. Only when a well-defined abscess is identified and the cytologic or bacteriologic studies absolutely confirm infection do the surgeons go in. In many cases the surgeon gives the patient a trial of intravenous antibiotics in the hopes that the abscess will resolve or in an attempt to reduce the infection around the abscess so that the wall of the collection "matures." A soggy parotid gland filled with purulent material is just not a great background for dissecting vital cranial nerves. The surgical approach—debridement, drainage, and preservation of normal parotid tissue—is vastly different than the philosophy of neoplasm removal in which a cuff of normal tissue is removed without violation of the lesion's capsule.

Notes

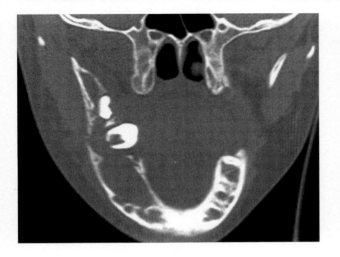
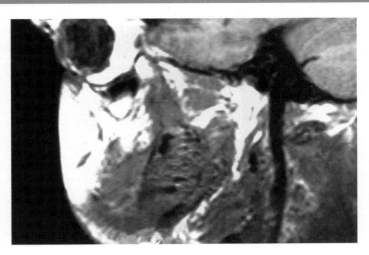
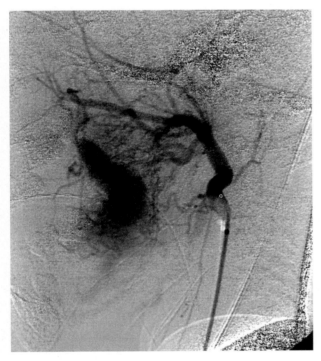

1. Are arteriovenous fistulas (AVFs) of the head and neck more common than true arteriovenous malformations?

2. What are the typical symptoms associated with facial AVFs?

3. What is the most common cause of AVFs of the head and neck?

4. What is the treatment for such AVFs?

Mandibular Arteriovenous Fistula

1. Yes.

2. Bruits, tinnitus, erythema, and swelling.

3. Trauma (especially carotid-cavernous fistulas, penetrating wounds to the neck).

4. Transvascular embolization and/or surgical ligation.

Reference

Halbach VV, Higashida RT, Hieshima GB, Hardin CW: Arteriovenous fistula of the internal maxillary artery: treatment with transarterial embolization, *Radiology* 168:443-445, 1988.

Cross-Reference

Neuroradiology: THE REQUISITES, pp 144-145.

Comment

This is a difficult case. The CT shows a lytic lesion of the mandible, and an arteriovenous malformation is not the first thing one should think of, given the CT appearance. The sagittal MRI is through the ascending ramus and body of the mandible, and one can see signal voids associated with the flowing blood channels. The arteriogram is from an internal maxillary artery injection, and one sees shunting of blood into a very large venous structure that is the origin of the "lytic bone lesion" identified on the CT. The patient had embolization of the mass, as well as ethanol sclerotherapy via a direct transcortical puncture of the mandible.

Every time I start to think about how I wish I did more invasive therapeutic procedures, along comes some disaster or anatomic variant that I have never seen before that could cause more damage to the patient than the cure. Remember that the meningolacrimal artery connects the middle meningeal artery (MMA) to the ophthalmic artery. If a large one is present, embolants placed into the MMA to embolize a meningioma can blind a patient. Remember the lateral mainstem or inferolateral trunk of the carotid artery—it can serve as a two-way street through which particles placed in internal maxillary artery branches can pass intracranially. Remember ethmoid to ophthalmic artery collaterals that can serve as conduits from the sinonasal cavity to the eye. Be careful. Ignorance may not be bliss!

Notes

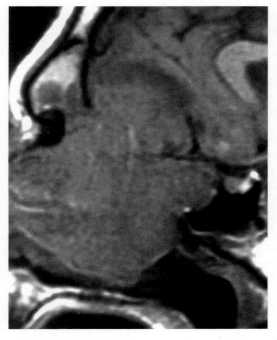
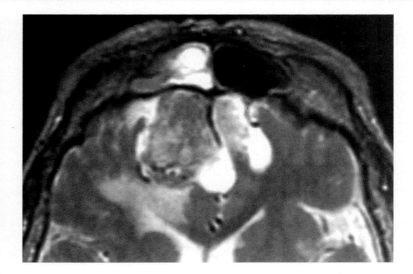

1. What criteria best distinguish dural invasion from dural reactivity secondary to a neoplasm?

2. What imaging features of a nasal skull base mass suggest olfactory neuroblastoma?

3. Describe the demographics of olfactory neuroblastomas.

4. Describe the Kadish staging of olfactory neuroblastomas.

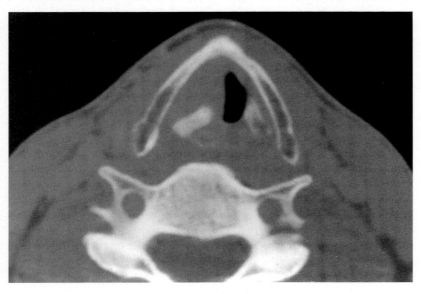

1. What does cartilaginous sclerosis imply?

2. What is the explanation for cartilaginous sclerosis without true invasion?

3. With which cartilage is the presence of sclerosis least valuable in suggesting tumoral invasion?

4. What other CT findings may be useful to diagnose cartilaginous invasion?

Dural Invasion by Olfactory Neuroblastoma

1. Enhancing dura greater than 5 mm in thickness, nodularity of the dural enhancement, enhancement or abnormal T2W signal intraparenchymally signifying transdural spread into the brain substance, and pial enhancement.

2. Calcification, cyst associated with the mass intracranially, epicenter at the cribriform plate, intermediate signal intensity on T2W scanning, and moderate contrast enhancement.

3. Two peaks are noted—in the 11- to 20-year-old group and in the 50- to 60-year-old group.

4. Stage A, confined to nasal cavity. Stage B, nasal cavity and paranasal sinuses. Stage C, beyond the nasal cavity and paranasal sinuses.

Reference

Eisen MD, Yousem DM, Montone KT, Kotapka MJ, Bigelow DC, Bilker WB, Loevner LA: Use of preoperative MR to predict dural, perineural, and venous sinus invasion of skull base tumors, *AJNR Am J Neuroradiol* 17:1937-1945, 1996.

Cross-Reference

Neuroradiology: THE REQUISITES, pp 373-374, 493.

Comment

Dural invasion by a tumor significantly decreases a patient's prognosis, with mean survival approximately 5 months. Patients without dural invasion but with a skull base mass have a 5-year prognosis that is 4 times better than those with dural invasion. Unfortunately, the dura may enhance because of inflammatory or "reactive" changes, which is why the criteria of nodular thickening, pial enhancement, or thickened dura greater than 5 mm are important to know. Perineural and perivascular invasion of skull base lesions are two other important findings that have great impact on prognosis.

More and more people are embracing the Dulguerov staging of esthesioneuroblastomas (olfactory neuroblastomas). T1 is nasal cavity and paranasal sinus disease (sparing upper ethmoids), T2 has extension to and erosion of the cribriform plate, T3 has extension to the orbit or protrusion into the anterior cranial fossa, and T4 shows brain invasion. Metastases to cervical lymph nodes, lungs, and bones are found in 20% of cases. This is a malignancy with a 5-year survival rate of about 50%. Unfortunately, the survival may be without an eye, with neurologic deficits, or with disfiguring surgical deformity secondary to invasion of the orbits, dura, or sinonasal cavity.

If calcification in a mass like this is present, consider olfactory neuroblastoma, inverted papilloma, chondrosarcoma of the nasal septum, osteosarcoma, and mucinous adenocarcinoma metastases.

Notes

Arytenoid Sclerosis Caused by Squamous Cell Carcinoma

1. Tumor is up to, if not through, the perichondrium of the cartilage.

2. An osteoblastic inflammatory reaction secondary to adjacent tumor.

3. The thyroid cartilage.

4. Disease through and through into the strap muscles (extralaryngeal tumor), serpiginous contour to the laryngeal cartilage, erosion of cartilage, and obliteration of medullary space of cartilage.

Reference

Becker M, Zbaren P, Delavelle J, Kurt AM, Egger C, Rufenacht DA, Terrier F: Neoplastic invasion of the laryngeal cartilage: reassessment of criteria for diagnosis at CT, *Radiology* 203: 521-532, 1997.

Zbaren P, Becker M, Lang H: Staging of laryngeal cancer: endoscopy, computed tomography and magnetic resonance versus histopathology, *Eur Arch Otorhinolaryngol Suppl* 1:S117-122, 1997.

Cross-Reference

Neuroradiology: THE REQUISITES, pp 399-403.

Comment

MRI has been found to be more sensitive (89% versus 66%) but less specific (94% versus 84%) than CT for cartilage invasion. MRI tends to be more accurate in evaluating cricoid and arytenoid cartilages, whereas CT is better for thyroid cartilage. However, no MRI or CT study has achieved greater than 80% accuracy for predicting thyroid cartilage invasion with cancer because of its propensity for reactive change from neighboring tumor and because of its variable ossification. However, one can generalize that the greater the degree of cartilaginous invasion (from perichondrial to intracartilaginous to extracartilaginous), the higher the rate of detectability. With MRI, one might see abnormal marrow signal and enhancement in cartilage purely as a result of reactive change. Similarly, one may see sclerosis and erosion of the cartilage on CT without invasion. Why should we care? In most hands, the presence of cartilage invasion precludes radiation therapy as the primary therapeutic modality and/or may predict radiation treatment failure. The potential for perichondritis in patients treated for cancer in the cartilage and concomitant airway collapse is devastating. In a similar vein, in most hands, voice conservation therapy is contraindicated with cartilaginous invasion (particularly the cricoid and arytenoid cartilages).

Notes

CASE 59

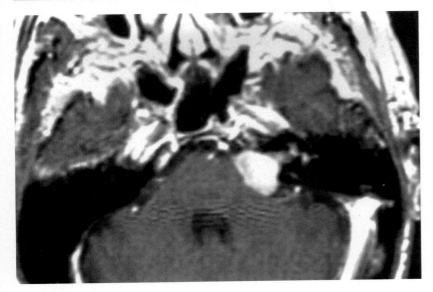

1. What is the unusual feature of this schwannoma?

2. What does the differential diagnosis of a contrast-enhancing mass in the cerebellopontine angle cistern include?

3. What percentage of acoustic (or vestibular) schwannomas are purely intracanalicular?

4. What are the criteria for neurofibromatosis type 2?

CASE 60

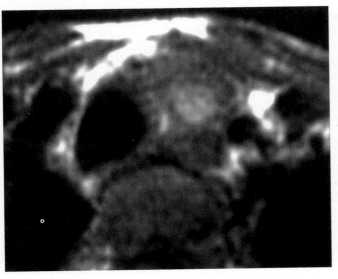
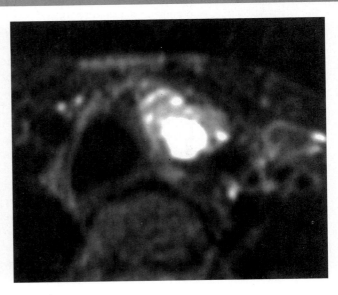

1. What are the most common causes of primary hyperparathyroidism?

2. What is the single best imaging choice to identify a parathyroid adenoma?

3. What percentage of newly diagnosed parathyroid adenomas are ectopic, and where do they occur?

4. What are the potential complications of parathyroid adenoma surgery?

Schwannoma Growing in the Cochlea and Vestibule

1. The lesion appears to grow into the cochlea, vestibule, and semicircular canals.

2. Schwannomas of the seventh and eighth nerve and occasionally the fifth nerve, meningiomas, exophytic brainstem gliomas, subarachnoid seeds on the nerves, desmoplastic medulloblastomas, and pial hemangioblastomas.

3. Twenty percent. (Around 65% are just extracanalicular.)

4. Bilateral vestibular schwannomas; or a first degree relative with neurofibromatosis type 2 and either one acoustic schwannoma or two of the following: nonacoustic schwannomas, neurofibromas, meningiomas, or gliomas.

Reference
Starshak RJ: Chromosome 22: a model with implications for diagnostic imaging, *AJR Am J Roentgenol* 167:315-324, 1996.

Cross-Reference
Neuroradiology: THE REQUISITES, p 347.

Comment
Neurofibromatosis type 2 is one of a number of diseases that has been linked to chromosome 22, including DiGeorge syndrome, Schindler disease, chronic myelogenous leukemia, Ewing's sarcoma, peripheral primitive neuroectodermal tumors, meningiomas, metachromatic leukodystrophy, and sporadic vestibular schwannomas. Neurofibromatosis type 2 is transmitted in an autosomal dominant fashion with greater than 90% penetrance. Over 50% of patients with neurofibromatosis type 2 also develop a meningioma in their lifetime. Cystic components to vestibular schwannomas are reported in 4% of cases, and they appear to have a faster growth rate than purely solid schwannomas.

If there were just cochlear and vestibular enhancement in this case, one would shift focus from the neoplastic category to the inflammatory lesions because labyrinthitis may cause this appearance (and labyrinthitis is a much more common entity in general than labyrinthine schwannomas). It is usually thought that "acoustic neuromas" are actually schwannomas of the vestibular nerves. The unusual aspect of this case is its extensive growth into the cochlea and the vestibule and even (subtle on this image) into the lateral semicircular canal. I guess this tumor just went wild and encapsulated all of the eighth nerve branches.

Notes

Parathyroid Adenoma

1. Parathyroid adenoma (80%), parathyroid hyperplasia (15%), multiple parathyroid adenomas (4%), and parathyroid carcinoma (1%).

2. Technetium Tc 99m sestamibi scanning.

3. Ten percent to 15% are ectopic. They may occur in the periesophageal, low cervical, or mediastinal locations. Intrathyroidal parathyroid adenomas may also occur.

4. Persistent hyperparathyroidism, hypoparathyroidism, injury to the recurrent laryngeal nerve causing vocal cord paralysis, and injuries to nearby blood vessels.

Reference
Gordon BM, Gordon L, Hoang K, Spicer KM: Parathyroid imaging with 99m Tc-sestamibi, *AJR Am J Roentgenol* 167: 1563-1568, 1996.

Cross-Reference
Neuroradiology: THE REQUISITES, p 443.

Comment
Many parathyroid surgeons do not believe that they need any imaging studies to find parathyroid adenomas in the neck because success rates of greater than 90% without imaging have been reported by experienced operators. Often it is an unsuccessful bilateral neck exploration in which the adenoma is ectopic that causes the surgeon to do a "peak and shriek" and run to the radiologist for help. Why not just get the imaging study, do a unilateral exploration, decrease operating room time, and play it safe? Money, or perhaps it is the heroic mentality. Surgeons *are* unanimous in supporting the need for imaging after a failed initial surgery. Regardless of whether you image primarily or after a failed surgery, what test is the best? I used to advocate ultrasound (cheap and effective and the clinicians cannot easily read it themselves), CT (nice to differentiate thyroid tissue from parathyroid lesions, goes to the mediastinum well), or MRI (adenomas are bright on T2W and enhance, and we make the most bucks on these studies) to search for a parathyroid adenoma. These days you just can't beat the sestamibi nuclear scintigraphy scan. It is cost effective, can tell a node from an adenoma (which the other studies usually cannot), can see into the mediastinum, and is reasonably specific. Why fight it? Throw the nukes guys a bone. This case is difficult because the scans do not show the thyroid gland, and the lesion was hemorrhagic. Give yourself partial credit if you said a degenerated hemorrhagic thyroid adenoma. Unfortunately, the clinical history was hypercalcemia, and it was a parathyroid adenoma.

Notes

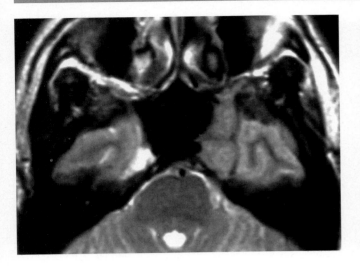
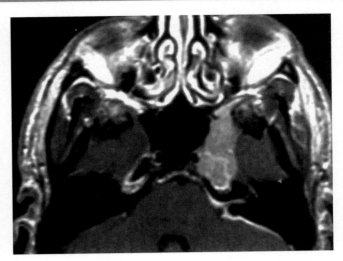
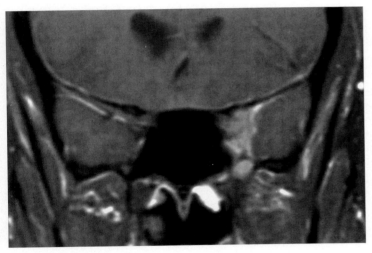

1. Along what cranial nerve is this lesion spreading?

2. What does the differential diagnosis include?

3. What type of lymphoma most commonly affects the dura?

4. What is the incidence of CNS involvement with sarcoidosis?

Dural Lymphoma

1. The fifth cranial nerve via the foramen rotundum.

2. Neurogenic tumors, meningioma, lymphoma, metastases, and dural plasmacytomas.

3. Non-Hodgkin's lymphoma (diffuse histiocytic type).

4. Fifteen percent.

Reference

Fukui MB, Meltzer CC, Kanal E, Smirniotopoulos JG: MR imaging of the meninges. Part II: neoplastic disease, *Radiology* 201:605-612, 1996.

Cross-Reference

Neuroradiology: THE REQUISITES, pp 74-75, 90-92.

Comment

This tumor appears to emanate from Meckel's cave, and one should consider fifth nerve lesions given this appearance. The finding that bodes against a schwannoma of the fifth nerve is the presence of dural enhancement extending around the cerebellum and into the internal auditory canal—a schwannoma would not do this, so one shifts to the possibilities of meningioma, lymphoma, and dural metastases, probably in that order.

The incidence of positive CSF cytology in tumors that have invaded the meninges is variable, with reported sensitivities of 63% for glioblastoma multiforme and 80% for non-CNS primary tumors, provided that three CSF samples are performed. MRI with gadolinium is a complementary study in most cases, with false negative rates reported at approximately 30%. Imaging studies do worse with lymphomatous and leukemic subarachnoid and dural spread than with other tumors. It seems that when the dura is infiltrated, as opposed to the pia or subarachnoid space, CSF cytology has a lower accuracy, but imaging has a better chance at detection.

Dural plasmacytomas occur as isolated lesions or as part of a plasma cell dyscrasia–myelomatous spectrum. Solitary craniocerebral plasmacytomas are eminently curable local masses that usually present as a result of headaches and meningeal irritation. They are unassociated with multiple myeloma and are a separate entity from metastatic multiple myeloma to the skull, yet they do represent a monoclonal proliferation of plasma cells. A monoclonal spike of immunoglobulin in the blood or urine may allow definitive distinction of the entity from meningioma, lymphoma, and sarcoidosis. Also in the differential diagnosis is a plasma cell granuloma—a polyclonal proliferation of plasma cells that looks just like the solitary craniocerebral plasmacytoma. Osseous plasmacytomas most commonly affect the parietal bone and skull base. The plasmacytoma is sensitive to radiotherapy.

Notes

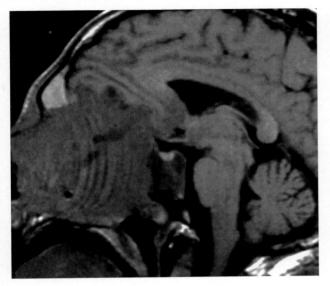
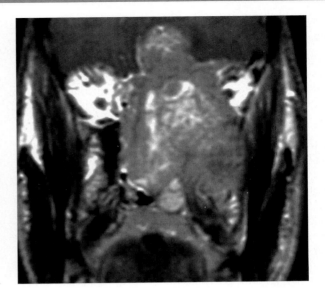

1. In which sinus do carcinomas occur most frequently?

2. What is the best way to distinguish between secretions and cancer in the sinonasal cavity?

3. Intracranial cysts are associated with what sinonasal neoplasm?

4. What is the significance of a lesion producing concavity of the perimuscular fat in the orbit without infiltration of that fat?

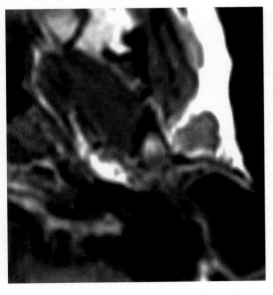
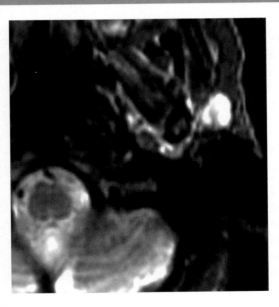

1. What are the demographics of oncocytomas?

2. What lesions in the parotid gland accumulate technetium Tc 99m pertechnetate?

3. What is the characteristic location of an oncocytoma?

4. What is the incidence of bilaterality in oncocytomas?

CASE 62

Sinonasal Undifferentiated Carcinoma

1. The maxillary sinus.

2. In general, gadolinium enhancement characteristics are the most reliable means. Contrast enhancement in a solid fashion is suggestive of tumor rather than inflammatory secretions, which enhance peripherally.

3. Olfactory neuroblastoma.

4. It usually means that the periorbita is intact and has successfully prevented intraorbital invasion.

Reference

Phillips CD, Futterer SF, Lipper MH, Levine PA: Sinonasal undifferentiated carcinoma: CT and MR imaging of an uncommon neoplasm of the nasal cavity, *Radiology* 202:477-480, 1997.

Cross-Reference

Neuroradiology: THE REQUISITES, pp 371-372.

Comment

Sinonasal undifferentiated carcinoma has a worse prognosis than squamous cell carcinoma, adenocarcinoma, or minor salivary gland cancers of the paranasal sinuses. It is highly aggressive, analogous to the anaplastic carcinoma of the thyroid gland. The tumors are large, grow quickly, and favor the ethmoid sinuses. Heterogeneous enhancement and early extension outside the paranasal sinuses into the brain and orbit are characteristic. At the upper nasal cavity—ethmoid region, the main differential diagnosis includes olfactory neuroblastoma (calcifications?), neuroendocrine tumor (low T2W intensity), lymphoepithelioma (bland looking), and adenocarcinoma (wood dust exposure). No specific imaging features are reported to distinguish this malignancy from others of the sinonasal cavity. Squamous cell carcinoma is the most common malignancy of the paranasal sinuses, accounting for approximately 80% of cases.

Another possibility for this case is a neuroendocrine tumor. Although the two most common sites reported for neuroendocrine tumors in the head and neck are the larynx-trachea and sinonasal cavity, I have only seen this tumor in the sinonasal cavity. Indium-111 octreotide scintigraphy has been able to diagnose some APUD tumors, including neuroendocrine tumors, carcinoid tumors, Merkel cell tumors, and paragangliomas.

The issues that should be addressed with any sinonasal cancer include involvement of (1) the orbit, (2) the skull base, (3) the dura, (4) the carotid artery, (5) nodal metastases, and (6) perineural extension. One must remember that aggressive-looking bone destruction can be present in the face of benign etiologies, including inverted papillomas, sinonasal polyposis, mycetomas, and pseudotumor of the sinus.

Notes

CASE 63

Oncocytoma of the Parotid Gland

1. The lesions occur in elderly individuals, most frequently in the parotid gland.

2. Warthin's tumors and oncocytomas.

3. In the superficial portion of the parotid gland over the masseter muscle.

4. Three percent to 7%.

Reference

San Pedro EC, Lorberboym M, Machac J, Som P, Shugar J: Imaging of multiple bilateral parotid gland oncocytomas, *Clin Nucl Med* 20:515-518, 1995.

Cross-Reference

Neuroradiology: THE REQUISITES, p 420.

Comment

One must remember that oncocytomas (oxyphilic adenomas) and Warthin's tumors are hot at ^{99m}Tc pertechnetate scintigraphy. This fact can help distinguish these two benign conditions from other masses in the parotid glands and, because they have little malignant potential, may influence therapy. The normal salivary gland tissue does concentrate the radiotracer, but the tumors show marked uptake against this background with less washout than normal glandular tissue. Warthin's tumors occur commonly in men and are frequently bilateral. They often have cystic regions. This particular case could easily have been a pleomorphic adenoma. The elderly age of the patient and the characteristic location of the lesion (pretragal or over the masseter) were the only clues to the correct diagnosis. I do not recommend suggesting this diagnosis because it is a relatively rare entity.

When faced with a solitary lesion in the nonparotid salivary glands, one should also not suggest a Warthin's tumor or an oncocytoma. These two tumors are relatively exclusive to the parotid gland. Instead, one should consider pleomorphic adenoma, monomorphic adenoma, myoepithelioma, hemangioma, or malignancies.

Notes

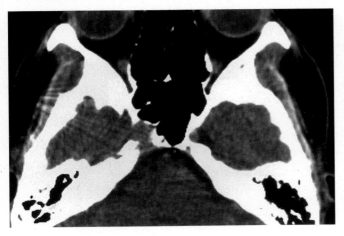
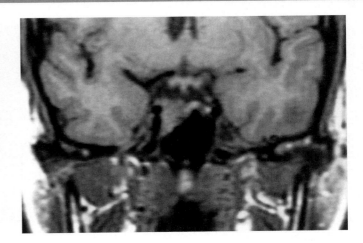

1. What is the prevalence of asymptomatic pituitary lesions in normal volunteers?

2. What are the three most common lesions of the cavernous sinus (the parasellar space)?

3. Describe the typical enhancement appearance of a pituitary microadenoma compared with the normal glandular tissue on scans at 2, 5, and 10 minutes after contrast administration.

4. What is the most common type of pituitary adenoma in prepubescent individuals?

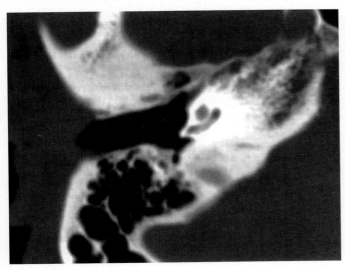
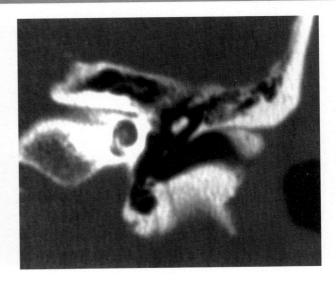

1. How many turns should be visible in the cochlea?

2. Before cochlear implant surgery, what normal structures should one evaluate on CT?

3. What is the potential value of MRI in the preoperative evaluation for cochlear implant?

4. Which inner ear congenital anomaly is the most common to cause sensorineural hearing loss?

Pituitary Adenoma

1. Six percent to 10% of normal adults have MRI findings consistent with pituitary adenomas.

2. Pituitary adenoma, schwannoma, and meningioma.

3. Initially the normal glandular tissue enhances more than the pituitary adenoma. At about 4 to 6 minutes after contrast enhancement, a crossover occurs in which the pituitary adenoma and the normal pituitary gland are isointense. After approximately 8 minutes the pituitary adenoma may show greater enhancement than the normal pituitary tissue.

4. Adrenocorticotropic hormone–secreting tumors.

Reference

Teramoto A, Hirakawa K, Sanno N, Osamura Y: Incidental pituitary lesions in 1000 unselected autopsy specimens, *Radiology* 193:161-164, 1994.

Cross-Reference

Neuroradiology: THE REQUISITES, p 313.

Comment

All that is hypointense in the pituitary gland is not a pituitary adenoma. One can find pituitary cysts, hyperplastic regions, infarcts, Rathke's cysts, and hemorrhages within the gland in asymptomatic individuals. Incidental (nonfunctioning) pituitary adenomas at autopsy occur in 2.7% to 22.5% of individuals. Beware of patients who have sellar masses and hypothyroidism. Pituitary hyperplasia caused by hypothyroidism producing avid TSH expression may simulate a pituitary adenoma. Also, do not overcall convexity of the upper margin of the gland or stalk deviation—these may be seen in normal individuals and are relatively common in pregnant women and in women who are hormonally active (which is not to imply that they are not "normal individuals"). Pituitary adenocarcinomas are reportable—I have never seen one.

Never forget a pituitary adenoma when you are evaluating a cavernous sinus, sellar, or perisellar mass. They are so common that they usually sneak in there just when you forget to mention them in a differential diagnosis. I have seen them grow as high as the top of the corpus callosum or grow down into the nasopharynx. Dynamic imaging suggests that scanning early on (<60 seconds) or after a slight delay (2.5 to 5 minutes) maximizes the contrast between normally enhancing pituitary tissue and delayed enhancing pituitary adenoma. I was fooled on this case based on the CT—I started thinking "cavernous sinus mass" and never considered a sellar etiology while interpreting the CT. The MRI snapped me back to reality.

Notes

Cochlear Stenosis before Cochlear Implant Caused by Labyrinthitis Ossificans

1. Two and one-half to 2¾ turns.

2. The cochlea and round window for patency, and the facial nerve, carotid artery, and jugular vein for their positions relative to the surgical approaches.

3. MRI may be more useful to evaluate for membranous/fibrous cochlear stenosis than CT, which is better for looking at bony cochlear stenosis.

4. Enlargement of the vestibular aqueduct.

Reference

Weissman JL: Hearing loss, *Radiology* 199:593-611, 1996.

Cross-Reference

Neuroradiology: THE REQUISITES, p 351.

Comment

Labyrinthitis ossificans usually occurs as a sequela of chronic labyrinthitis, meningitis, or trauma with fibrous and/or bony obliteration of the inner ear structures. Primary luetic labyrinthitis or spread from middle ear infections may cause labyrinthitis obliterans as well. Cogan's syndrome (interstitial keratitis and audiovestibular dysfunction) is characterized by the obliteration of intralabyrinthine spaces. This may be due to calcification or fibrous tissue of the lateral semicircular canal and/or vestibule. Inner ear labyrinth ossification is easily seen with CT (if you know to look for it), but if there is fibrous obliteration it will be better seen on high resolution T2W MRI scanning. The deficit is usually sensorineural hearing loss. Otosclerosis—an entirely different entity in which there is replacement of dense bone with spongiotic, lucent bone—also causes sensorineural hearing loss.

Notes

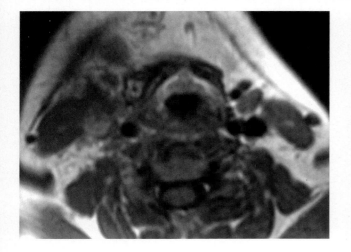
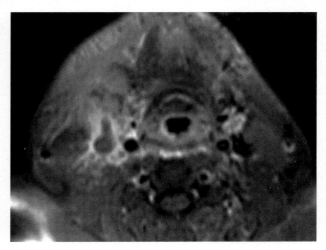
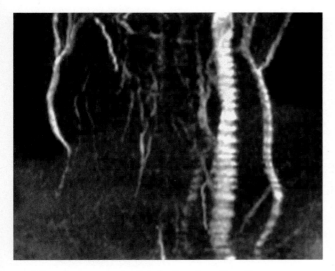

1. To what space is this lesion localized?

2. What are the most common causes of inflammatory disease to affect the carotid space?

3. In what ways are thromboses of the blood vessel different in their signal intensity characteristics than intraparenchymal hematomas?

4. Define postanginal sepsis.

Internal Jugular Vein Thrombophlebitis

1. The carotid space.

2. Lymphadenitis, jugular thrombophlebitis, and pharyngitis.

3. There is often lamination of thrombus, no hemosiderin deposition, and a delay in the evolution of the hemorrhagic blood products.

4. It is similar to Ludwig's angina and is an infection of the oral cavity or oropharynx that spreads directly into the mediastinum or via thrombophlebitis and pulmonary emboli.

Reference

Poe LB, Manzione JV, Wasenko JJ, Kellman RM: Acute internal jugular vein thrombosis associated with pseudoabscess of the retropharyngeal space, *AJNR Am J Neuroradiol* 16:892-896, 1995.

Cross-Reference

Neuroradiology: THE REQUISITES, p 431.

Comment

The usual differential diagnosis of jugular vein thrombophlebitis is a neck abscess. In the former, the jugular vein is usually increased in size, and there is a history of catheter insertion, malignancy, hypercoagulable state, leukemia/lymphoma, or drug use with jugular venous injections. Slow flow in the jugular vein may cause high signal intensity on T1W scans and may simulate thrombosis. Beware of this potential pitfall. Do a magnetic resonance venogram (MRV)! Unfortunately, if there is hyperintense clot on the T1W MRI, a time of flight MRV may show "flow" in the vein that is actually subacute clot. You would have to do a phase contrast MRV to completely sort this out. It helps to know these nuances when you are running the scanner. The enhancement around the clotted vein in this case is indicative of superimposed infection, and the patient was septic.

Edema and enhancement of the parapharyngeal and retropharyngeal space may occur in association with internal jugular vein thrombophlebitis. The fluid density in the retropharyngeal space may simulate a retropharyngeal abscess, phlegmon, suppurative adenitis, or cellulitis. It has been postulated that the retropharyngeal edema comes from transudation of fluid from the posterior pharyngeal venous plexus, interstitial fluid, and lymphatic engorgement.

Notes

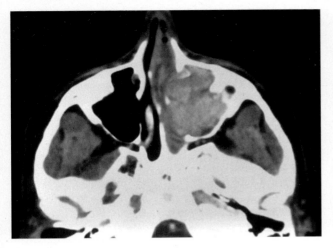 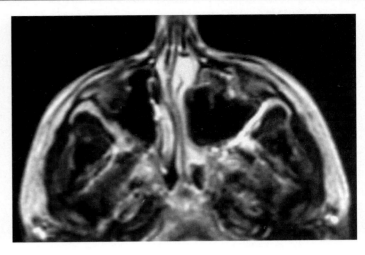

1. True or false: Air-fluid levels are common in fungal sinusitis.

2. How can fungal sinusitis simulate normal aeration on MRI scanning?

3. Describe the typical patient with acute fulminant *Aspergillus* infection.

4. Describe the typical patient who has a mycetoma.

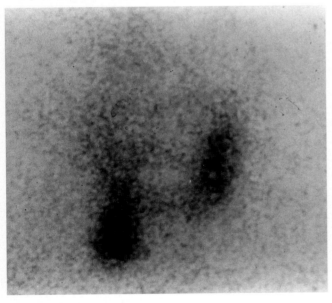 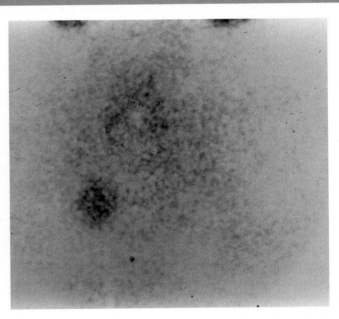

1. What radiotracer has been injected, and what is the difference between the two scintigrams performed?

2. What are the potential false positive results with sestamibi scanning?

3. How accurate is sestamibi scanning for diagnosing parathyroid hyperplasia?

4. What are the advantages of sestamibi scanning over thallium scanning?

Fungal Sinusitis

1. False.

2. Often the fungus shows decreased signal intensity on both T1W and T2W scanning, making it look like air within the sinus rather than dense, calcified, manganese-encrusted fungi.

3. This typically occurs in an immune-comprised individual who has diminished white blood cells.

4. This usually occurs in an immune-competent individual who has had recent surgery or radiotherapy, or who has a background of allergic sinusitis. Marijuana smokers may have an increased risk of developing fungus balls.

Reference

Ashdown BC, Tien RD, Felsberg GJ: Aspergillosis of the brain and paranasal sinuses in immunocompromised patients: CT and MR imaging findings, *AJR Am J Roentgenol* 162:155-159, 1994.

Cross-Reference

Neuroradiology: THE REQUISITES, pp 366-368.

Comment

What happened to the opacified sinus between the CT and the MRI? It's still there; it's just that fungi and/or inspissated secretions may have a signal void on a T2W MRI sequence. Even on the T1W and post-gadolinium scans, this patient's sinus looked dark. Some believe this is due to calcification; some think that manganese accumulation in the fungus is to blame. Certainly one can see calcifications in aspergillomas, but drechsleria grew out of this patient's cultures.

Aspergillus fumigatus is the usual pathogen to cause intracranial disseminated mycotic infections in immune-compromised individuals (AIDS patients, patients on immunosuppressive drugs, leukemics, dialysis patients, intravenous drug abusers, transplant patients, and so on). Once the brain is involved the prognosis is pretty poor, with the potential for abscesses, infarcts, and meningeal spread. Mycotic aneurysms and intracranial hematomas may also occur as the fungi cause intraluminal obstruction. Low signal intensity rings on T2W scans are often seen with *Aspergillus* abscesses, just like the sinusitis may be dark on T2W scans. In my experience, the worst cases of fungal infections spreading intracranially have actually been due to invasive mucormycosis, not *Aspergillus*. Frankly, I would not want either of them eating away at my sinuses.

Notes

Parathyroid Adenoma on Sestamibi Scanning

1. Technetium Tc 99m pertechnetate sestamibi has been injected, and the second scan is delayed 2 hours after the first scan.

2. Thyroid masses, bronchogenic/tracheal masses, and other head and neck cancers.

3. Approximately 60% accurate.

4. Because the technetium has a higher photon energy, it is able to penetrate the mediastinum better, allowing one to see ectopic parathyroid adenomas more clearly. Additionally, the signal to noise is better. Finally, one can use single tracer imaging rather than having to rely on subtraction imaging from technetium pertechnetate or iodine-123 scans of the thyroid gland.

Reference

Lee VS, Wilkinson RH Jr, Leigh GS Jr, Coogan AC, Coleman RE: Hyperparathyroidism in high-risk surgical patients: evaluation with double-phase technetium-99m sestamibi imaging, *Radiology* 197:627-634, 1995.

Cross-Reference

Neuroradiology: THE REQUISITES, p 443.

Comment

Technetium pertechnetate sestamibi scanning has largely replaced the thallium-technetium pertechnetate subtraction technique for imaging adenomas because it is 95% accurate. It is unclear whether the concentration of sestamibi in parathyroid adenomas is on the basis of high mitochondrial concentration or on a hypervascularity basis. To determine hyperplasia of the glands as a cause of first degree or second degree hyperparathyroidism, no agent is very good—typical treatment is to resect three and one-half glands and hope for the best. Sestamibi has accuracy rates for adenomas in the 95% range, but for hyperplasia it is only 64% sensitive (although it has a percentage in the high 90s for specificity). Of course, the larger the gland, the higher the rate of detection. The accuracy rate of ultrasound and CT for detecting parathyroid gland hyperplasia is only approximately 30% to 40% and is in the 75% to 85% range for detecting adenomas. In evaluating a patient for a parathyroid adenoma or parathyroid hyperplasia, a thyroid mass is significant because of the possibility of intrathyroidal parathyroid adenomas. Also, in patients with hyperparathyroidism there can be medullary carcinoma of the thyroid gland as part of a combined multiple endocrine neoplasia syndrome.

In patients who have failed initial operations for primary hyperparathyroidism, 70% to 75% of adenomas are found in the perithyroid location.

Notes

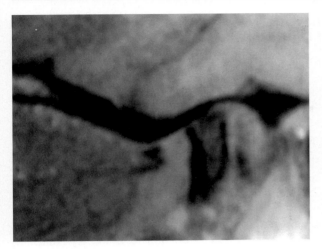 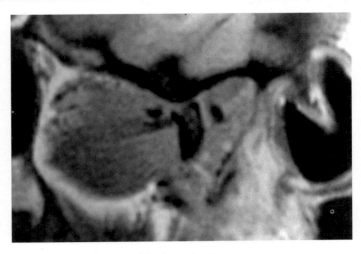

1. What are the most common inflammatory arthritides of the temporomandibular joint?

2. How does one distinguish rheumatoid arthritis of the temporomandibular joint from osteoarthritis?

3. Describe the locations of joint effusions in the temporomandibular joint.

4. True or false: Rheumatoid arthritis of the temporomandibular joint is associated with a higher rate of meniscal perforation than osteoarthritis.

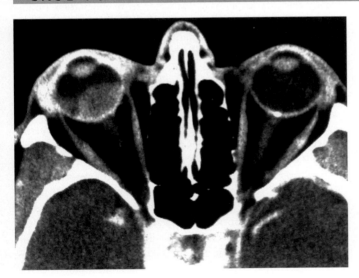

1. What is the most common primary malignant neoplasm of the choroid?

2. What are the unique signal intensity features of melanin-containing melanomas of the orbit?

3. If calcification within an ocular mass is present, what should one consider in the differential diagnosis?

4. In a child who has a mass that is hyperintense on T1W scans in the globe, what should one consider?

Rheumatoid Arthritis of the Temporomandibular Joint

1. Rheumatoid arthritis, psoriatic arthritis, ankylosing spondylitis, gout, and septic arthritis.

2. Absence of bony sclerosis and hyperostosis; predominance of erosion; and synovial thickening.

3. There are superior and inferior compartments to the temporomandibular joint on either side of the anterior band of the meniscus. Similar findings are present posteriorly.

4. True.

References

Larheim TA, Smith HJ, Aspestrand F: Temporomandibular joint abnormalities associated with rheumatic disease: comparison between MR imaging and arthrotomography, *Radiology* 183:221-226, 1992.

Smith HJ, Larheim TA, Aspestrand F: Rheumatic and nonrheumatic disease in the temporomandibular joint: gadolinium-enhanced MR imaging, *Radiology* 185:229-234, 1992.

Cross-Reference

Neuroradiology: THE REQUISITES, pp 424-427.

Comment

This case shows erosions of the mandibular condyle, fragmentation of a degenerated meniscus, narrowing of the joint without bony eburnation, and synovial thickening. Range of motion is good. Rheumatoid arthritis affects the temporomandibular joint in about 50% of individuals. Condylar destruction or erosions (82%), disk disruption, effusions (23%), disk fragmentation or perforation (23%), and synovial thickening (73%) may be present on the MRI. In the late phase of rheumatoid arthritis of the temporomandibular joint, bony or fibrous ankylosis with no intervening tissue may be present (23%). Contrast enhancement of synovial tissue, articular surfaces, menisci, and/or synovial effusions of the temporomandibular joint may be seen with the inflammatory arthritides.

Another site of rheumatoid arthritis in the head and neck is the cricoarytenoid joint. Limitation of motion and swelling of the joint may occur that may affect voice. Fusion of the joint may cause permanent voice changes. Look for erosions and edema on CT. Destruction by rheumatoid disease may simulate chondronecrosis from other causes (radiation, relapsing polychondritis, neoplasm).

Notes

Choroidal Melanoma on Right, Drusen of Optic Nerve on Left

1. Melanoma.

2. Melanin is usually bright on T1W scans, and there is intermediate to low intensity on T2W scans.

3. Retinoblastoma, choroidal hemangiomas, choroidal osteomas, *Toxocara* infections, astrocytic hamartomas, and chronic retinal or choroidal detachments.

4. If the globe is small, one should consider persistent hyperplastic primary vitreous. If the globe is of normal size with calcification, one should consider retinoblastoma.

Reference

Hosten N, Bornfeld N, Wassmuth R, Lemke AJ, Sander B, Bechrakis NE, Felix R: Uveal melanoma: detection of extraocular growth with MR imaging and US, *Radiology* 202:61-67, 1997.

Cross-Reference

Neuroradiology: THE REQUISITES, p 287.

Comment

Ocular melanomas can be found in the iris (6%), ciliary body (9%), and choroid (85%). These three structures constitute the uveal tract that contains melanocytes, from which these tumors develop. Melanomas are second only to metastases as the most common intraocular malignancy in adults. Whites are affected over 8 times more frequently than African Americans. Melanomas may grow along the optic nerve, into the subarachnoid space, or outside the uveal tract and globe (10% to 15% of cases). MRI has recently been shown to be more sensitive and specific than high frequency ultrasound in detecting extraocular growth. This finding has dramatic prognostic implications, decreasing 5-year prognoses to the 40% range. Hematogenous dissemination leads to liver metastases most commonly.

Ultrasound is the most sensitive means for detecting optic nerve head drusen. They are often bilateral and may run in families. They are usually asymptomatic, seen as a fleck of calcification at the optic nerve head insertion to the globe on CT (along with the other "senile" calcifications of muscular tendinous insertions). Included in the differential diagnosis are retinoblastoma, astrocytic hamartoma (seen in tuberous sclerosis and neurofibromatosis), and choroidal osteomas, but these are not so exquisitely located right in the nerve head. The optic nerve head may appear swollen and simulate papilledema. Elsewhere in the globe the presence of drusen may be indicative of a retinal degenerative disease and may influence vision.

Notes

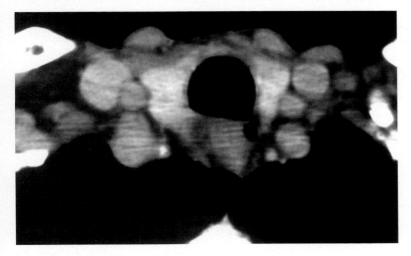

1. What is the correct name for the area of weakness in the cricopharyngeus muscle?

2. Differentiate a Zenker's diverticulum from a Killian-Jamieson diverticulum.

3. What are the classic symptoms of a Zenker's diverticulum?

4. The cricopharyngeus is a portion of what part of the head and neck?

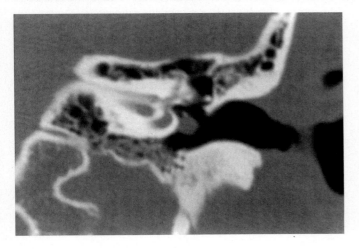 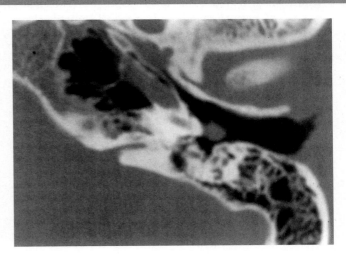

1. What is the most common cause of pulsatile tinnitus in a neurologist's practice?

2. What is the critical differential diagnosis of a glomus tympanicum tumor?

3. What is the difference between objective and subjective tinnitus?

4. Near what structure does a glomus tympanicum usually reside?

Zenker's Diverticulum of the Esophagus

1. Killian's (Killian-Jamieson) dehiscence.

2. Zenker's is a true diverticulum of the mucosa, whereas a Killian-Jamieson diverticulum is due to a muscular dehiscence between the oblique and longitudinal cricopharyngeus fibers.

3. Dysphagia and odynophagia, with delayed vomiting of undigested food in an elderly individual.

4. The hypopharynx.

Reference
Rubesin SE: The pharynx: structural disorders, *Radiol Clin North Am* 32:1083-1101, 1994.

Cross-Reference
Neuroradiology: THE REQUISITES, p 393.

Comment
Zenker's diverticulum is a herniation of mucosa through the upper esophageal sphincter that occurs as a result of long-term pressure elevation at that site. Premature closure of the upper esophageal sphincter or mistiming of the normal swallowing manometrics may lead to the diverticulum. Gastroesophageal reflux, which may put the upper esophageal sphincter into spasm, is a frequent finding in patients with this disorder. Lateral pharyngeal pouches occur higher than Zenker's diverticula in the upper hypopharynx at the thyrohyoid membrane level.

Who should get credit—Friedrich Albert von Zenker, a German pathologist (1825-1898); Gustav Killian, a German laryngologist (1860-1921); or Jamieson (unknown stats)? Better check the *Gastrointestinal Radiology: THE REQUISITES* volume for that information!

Notes

Glomus Tympanicum

1. Benign intracranial hypertension (pseudotumor cerebri).

2. Aberrance of the internal carotid artery.

3. With objective tinnitus both the patient and the examiner can hear the tinnitus. This is usually highly predictive of a vascular lesion as opposed to subjective tinnitus. With subjective tinnitus only the patient hears the sound.

4. The cochlear promontory.

Reference
Baguley DM, Irving RM, Hardy DG, Harada T, Moffat DA: Audiological findings in glomus tumors, *Br J Audiol* 28:291-297, 1994.

Sismanis A, Butts FM, Hughes GB: Objective tinnitus in benign intracranial hypertension: an update, *Laryngoscope* 100:33-36, 1990.

Cross-Reference
Neuroradiology: THE REQUISITES, p 344.

Comment
There are innumerable causes of pulsatile tinnitus. I was stunned to learn that benign intracranial hypertension (pseudotumor cerebri) was the most common one reported in the neurology literature. This disease is seen in young women, most commonly with a higher rate in black and obese patients who complain of headaches, hearing loss, and associated visual loss. One must consider arterial sources of pulsatile tinnitus (arteriovenous malformations, aneurysms, aberrancies, atherosclerosis), venous lesions (high jugular bulbs, emissary veins), neoplastic causes (glomus tumors), inflammatory lesions (cholesteatomas, cholesterol granulomas, otosclerosis), and other normal anatomic variants. Remember that otoscopy cannot distinguish between glomus tympanicum tumors and glomus jugulare tumors. Here is where the radiologist can help.

Of paragangliomas, carotid body tumors are more common than glomus jugulare tumors, which are more common than glomus tympanicum tumors, which are more common than glomus vagale tumors. They are more frequent in women. Despite their hypervascularity, glomus tympanicum tumors are small enough so that blood loss during resection via a tympanotomy is rarely an issue. For other paragangliomas, preoperative angiography with embolization is advised.

Notes

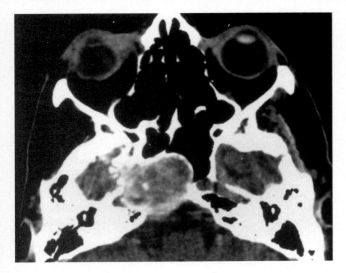

1. What does the differential diagnosis of this lesion include?

2. What is the best study to distinguish these entities?

3. What defines a giant aneurysm?

4. Are giant calcified aneurysms more or less likely to bleed than noncalcified, moderately sized (0.7 to 2 cm) aneurysms?

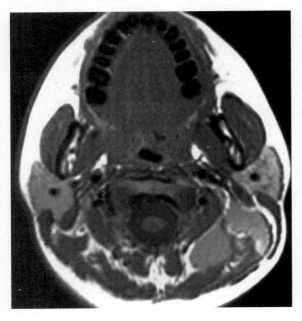 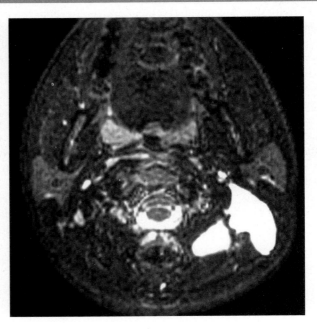

1. What are the typical locations of this lesion in the head and neck?

2. What syndromes are associated with a higher incidence of cystic hygromas?

3. Why may cystic hygromas be bright on T1W MRI scans?

4. Differentiate cystic hygromas from branchial cleft cysts.

Giant Aneurysm

1. Chordoma, chondrosarcoma, meningioma, cholesterol granuloma, and giant aneurysm.

2. Angiography (aneurysm seen or vessel occluded, meningioma fed by dural branches, chondrosarcoma relatively hypervascular, chordoma relatively hypovascular).

3. Size over 2.5 cm.

4. Less likely. (But I still wouldn't want one in my head!)

Reference

Love MHS, Bell KE: Giant aneurysm of the intrapetrous carotid artery presenting as a cerebellopontine angle mass, *Clin Radiol* 51:587-588, 1996.

Cross-Reference

Neuroradiology: THE REQUISITES, p 325.

Comment

I love these kinds of great teaching cases in which the importance of considering a potentially life-threatening lesion when faced with an unusual-looking scan can be emphasized. This ranks up there with the aberrant intrapetrous internal carotid artery. Petrous carotid artery aneurysms are very rare, and most are pseudoaneurysms caused by trauma, infection, or iatrogenic mishaps. The petrous carotid is very closely associated with the eustachian tube, separated only by a few layers of adventitia and cartilage. Therefore bleeding into the ear or nose can occur with petrous carotid aneurysms. Once the aneurysm is over 2.5 cm in size, it is called a giant aneurysm, and giant aneurysms not uncommonly calcify, partially thrombose, or even occlude.

On MRI giant aneurysms with thrombosis have palisading layers of high and low signal intensity from blood products of variable ages. It is important to try to assess for patency, with the caveat that deoxyhemoglobin may simulate flow voids on some pulse sequences. Methemoglobin may confound the issue on T1W scans and a time of flight MRA because it may appear bright on both scans. Therefore a phase contrast MRA may be of some value in evaluating giant aneurysms because even high signal intensity subacute clot does not show flow signal on the phase contrast MRA.

Notes

Cystic Hygroma of the Neck

1. In the posterior neck and in the lower neck extending to the axilla.

2. Turner's syndrome, Noonan's syndrome, and fetal alcohol syndrome.

3. Possibly because of trauma/hemorrhage, lymph, or high protein fluid.

4. Cystic hygromas are typically posterior to the sternocleidomastoid muscle, multiloculated, in children less than 2 years old, infiltrative, and multicompartmental.

Reference

Mancuso AA, Dillon WP: The neck, *Radiol Clin North Am* 27:407-434, 1989.

Cross-Reference

Neuroradiology: THE REQUISITES, pp 404-405.

Comment

The classic story for a cystic hygroma is a lesion present at birth (50%) or before age 2 years (90%) found in the posterior neck. It is usually compressible. I have also seen these lesions in the tongue, floor of mouth, parapharyngeal space, and orbit, presenting as large cystic spaces filled with fluid that is bright on T1W and T2W scans. Fluid-fluid levels (presumably as a result of hemorrhage into chylous or hyperproteinaceous material) may be present, but I have never seen air-fluid levels.

Cystic hygromas may extend into the axilla, entangle the brachial plexus, and dive into the upper mediastinum (10% of cases). The deep cervical space fascia is not respected by this lesion, and it insinuates aggressively. Whereas the signal may be variable on T1W scans, it is invariably bright on T2W scans. The multiseptated appearance and posterior location of the lesion typically gives the diagnosis away. In an infant the lesion is a "gimme." A teratoma is in the differential diagnosis when the mass is diffusely infiltrative. In an adult, sarcomas may appear similar but usually enhance.

Patients with Turner's syndrome have an XO genotype, a female phenotype, short stature, webbed necks, coarctation of the aorta and/or cardiac defects, and rudimentary gonadal development. Noonan's syndrome is the male phenotype of Turner's syndrome, with short stature, webbing of the neck, heart valve anomalies, and low-set ears.

Notes

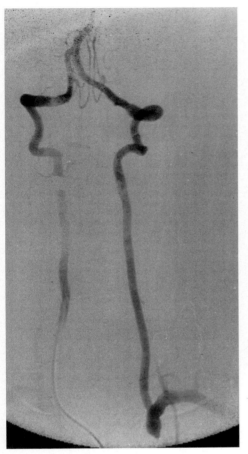 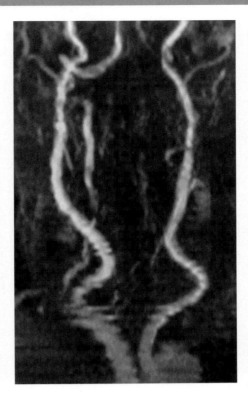 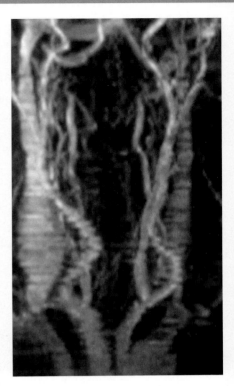

1. What is the usual cause of this angiographic finding?

2. Which arm of this patient will feel weak when at exercise?

3. Name three vasculopathies that may affect the proximal supraaortic vessels.

4. What is the typical injection rate and total volume used for a dominant vertebral artery arteriogram?

Subclavian Steal

1. Atherosclerosis of the proximal subclavian artery.

2. The left arm.

3. Choose three of the following: Takayasu's arteritis, temporal arteritis, fibromuscular dysplasia, polyarteritis nodosa, Wegener's granulomatosis, and Marfan syndrome.

4. Ranges obviously will vary, but the rate is usually 4 to 6 ml per second, and total volume is usually 7 to 10 ml.

References

Drutman J, Gyorke A, Davis WL, Turski PA: Evaluation of subclavian steal with two-dimensional phase-contrast and two-dimensional time-of-flight MR angiography, *AJNR Am J Neuroradiol* 15:1642-1646, 1994.

Cross-Reference

Neuroradiology: THE REQUISITES, p 109.

Comment

Subclavian steal affects the left arm more than the right, possibly because of the anatomy of the aortic arch branches with an innominate artery on the right side. Usual symptoms are arm fatigue with exercise, but patients may be asymptomatic unless they have concomitant atherosclerotic disease of the other cervical arteries. If a patient does have CNS symptoms, they usually manifest as dizziness and/or paresthesias in the affected arm. The diagnosis is often easily made by comparing blood pressures of the two arms and by noticing a delay in and reduction of strength in the pulse on the stealing side as compared with that on the healthy side. Risk factors for subclavian steal include the usual atherosclerotic ones, but baseball pitchers, cricket bowlers, people using crutches, and volleyball players are also at risk.

The figure in the middle and the figure on the right are nice demonstrations of how you can play with saturation pulses to demonstrate directional flow. The difference between the two scans is that saturation pulses were placed for inferior to superior flow in the figure in the middle, whereas no saturation pulses were placed in the figure on the right. The left vertebral artery is seen when no saturation pulses have been applied but not when the superior saturation pulse has been applied, suggesting retrograde flow down the vertebral artery—thus the classic "steal" phenomenon. You can do the same thing with phase contrast MRA, in which you can encode direction (and velocity) if you so desire. You have to be able to figure this case out when you see a flow void on the spin echo scan but no flow on your traditional superiorly saturated MRA.

Notes

CASE 76

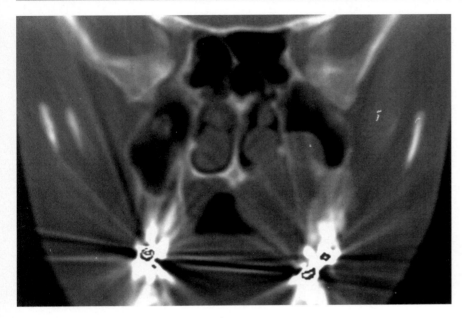

1. Name the bones of the hard palate.
2. In the hard palate, are benign or malignant lesions of the minor salivary glands more common?
3. Describe the T staging for oral cavity cancers.
4. What factors correlate with survival with malignant hard palate tumors?

CASE 77

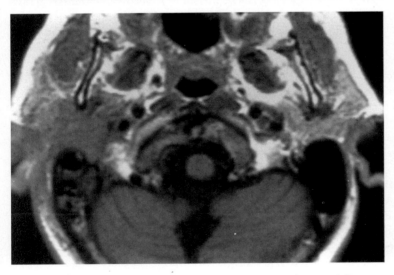 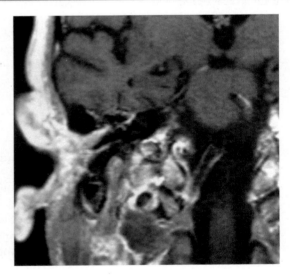

1. What two nerves are susceptible to perineural spread from a parotid space malignancy?
2. What is the most common salivary gland malignancy in children?
3. What is the most common malignancy of the lacrimal gland?
4. Which malignancy of the parotid gland has the highest rate of hematogenous metastases?

Mucoepidermoid Carcinoma of the Hard Palate

1. The palatine bones, the maxilla, and the pterygoid processes of the sphenoid bone.

2. Malignant lesions are more common (78% versus 22%, with adenoid cystic carcinoma the most common histologic type).

3. T1 tumor—2 cm or less in size; T2 tumor—greater than 2 cm but less than or equal to 4 cm in size; T3 tumor—greater than 4 cm in size; and T4 tumor—invading adjacent structures outside the oral cavity, including skin, cortical bone, soft tissues in the neck, and extrinsic muscles of the tongue.

4. Higher histologic grade, larger size, and positive surgical margins are independently associated with worse prognosis.

Reference

Beckhardt RN, Weber RS, Zane R, Garden AS, Wolf P, Carrillo R, Luna MA: Minor salivary gland tumors of the palate: clinical and pathologic correlates of outcome, *Laryngoscope* 105:1155-1160, 1995.

Cross-Reference

Neuroradiology: THE REQUISITES, pp 421-422.

Comment

Fifty percent of intraoral minor salivary gland tumors occur in the hard palate. Of benign tumors, pleomorphic adenomas constitute around 90%, and monomorphic adenomas comprise the remainder. From most to least common, adenoid cystic carcinomas, adenocarcinomas, and mucoepidermoid carcinomas account for malignancies. The radiologist must search for bony destruction, perineural invasion, and sinonasal infiltration to assist in surgical planning and prognostication. With clean surgical margins, 5-year survival is greater than 90%. Remember, however, that the adenoid cystic cancer can recur decades down the road with perineural spread, so chasing the fifth cranial nerve may be the end game in this region.

Note that the hard palate under the left inferior turbinate is destroyed in this case. This is the clearest indication that this lesion is not a benign maxillary sinus, odontogenic, or fibroosseous lesion. The region of the greater and lesser palatine canals is seen on the right side between the maxillary antrum and the nasal cavity inferiorly. That area is invaded on the left side, so infiltration of these branches of the maxillary nerve must be suspected. Note also the significant dental amalgam artifact. On MRI the artifact associated with dental fillings degrades the images to a lesser extent than on CT.

Notes

Squamous Cell Carcinoma of the Parotid Gland Extending up the Seventh Cranial Nerve

1. The fifth cranial nerve and the seventh cranial nerve.

2. Mucoepidermoid carcinoma.

3. Adenoid cystic carcinoma.

4. Adenoid cystic carcinoma.

Reference

Kane WJ, McCaffrey TV, Olsen KD, Lewis JE: Primary parotid malignancies, *Arch Otolaryngol Head Neck Surg* 117:307-315, 1991.

Cross-Reference

Neuroradiology: THE REQUISITES, p 338.

Comment

That squamous cell carcinoma can occur primarily in the parotid gland is always a source of angst for the head and neck surgeon. The surgeon must look arduously for a skin or aerodigestive mucosal primary malignancy to ensure that this is indeed a primary parotid squamous cell carcinoma and not a nodal metastases. It is thought that squamous metaplasia from columnar ductal lining cells accounts for the possibility of squamous malignancies here. In any case these lesions do poorly, and perineural spread (as in this case) is predictable. Facial nerve palsies present with parotid malignancies in 16% of cases—most parotid malignancies present as painless asymptomatic lumps. Squamous cell carcinoma ranks behind mucoepidermoid carcinoma, adenoid cystic carcinoma, adenocarcinoma, and acinic cell carcinoma in the parotid gland.

The axial scan nicely demonstrates the low intensity tumor in the right parotid gland making a posterior turn into the stylomastoid foramen, the egress of the facial nerve from the skull. If you look on the enhanced coronal scan medial to the dark mastoid tip, you see a very thick structure extending vertically into the temporal bone. This indeed is the thick enhancing descending intramastoid portion of the facial nerve encased with tumor.

Notes

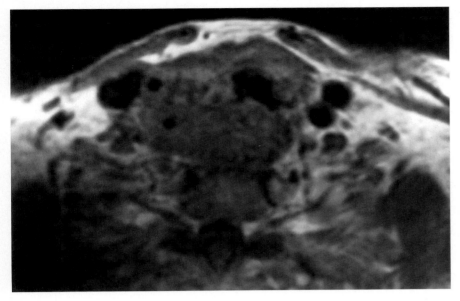

1. What is the best predictor of carotid invasion by tumor?

2. With which tumors is the criterion above least and most accurate?

3. Which affects the carotid artery most commonly—the primary tumor or nodal metastases?

4. Why is carotid encasement important to recognize?

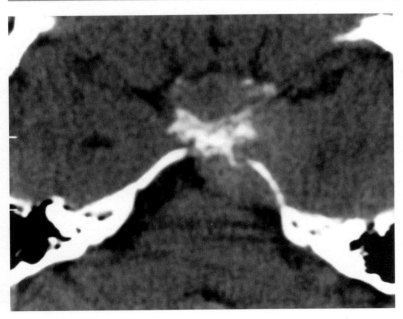

1. What is the significance of carotid encasement by cavernous sinus meningiomas?

2. How often do pituitary adenomas extend into the parasellar space?

3. Which tumor bleeds more frequently, an adenoma or a meningioma?

4. What other structures, besides the cavernous carotid artery, should be evaluated in patients who have parasellar meningiomas?

Carotid Encasement by Nodal Metastases from Lung Primary

1. Involvement of greater than 270 degrees around the circumference of the vessel.

2. Least accurate with chordomas, most accurate with squamous cell carcinomas.

3. It is very close, but primary tumors have the edge.

4. It is a bad prognostic sign, it may render the patient inoperable, and it may necessitate that the patient undergo balloon occlusion testing prior to resection to see if the carotid can be removed with the extirpation of the tumor.

Reference

Yousem DM, Hatabu H, Hurst RW, Seigerman HM, Montone KT, Weinstein GS, Hayden RE, Goldberg AN, Bigelow DC, Kotapka MJ: Carotid artery invasion by head and neck masses: prediction with MR imaging, *Radiology* 195:715-720, 1995.

Cross-Reference

Neuroradiology: THE REQUISITES, pp 432-433.

Comment

Only 5% to 20% of patients undergoing radical neck dissection for squamous cell carcinoma have carotid artery invasion, but the prognosis for patients who have this finding is dismal. One-year survival rates between 0% and 44% with high local and distant recurrence rates are often cited in the literature. When the carotid artery is ligated or resected, perioperative morbidity includes strokes (13% to 38% of cases), carotid rupture, abscess formation, and fistulas. Carotid rupture preoperatively or postoperatively may also be associated with prior irradiation. Thus it is important to accurately predict the presence of carotid invasion. Using the 270 degree criterion, MRI's sensitivity for predicting inoperable carotid encasement is 100% (11/11). The specificity is 85.2% (29/34), and accuracy is 88.9% (40/45). False positive cases occur most commonly in the cavernous carotid artery and with chordomas.

In this case, one might worry about a thyroid or upper esophageal malignancy as the source of this tumor. However, in addition to thinking about the lesion as a manifestation of the primary site in the neck, one must always consider adenopathy. Paratracheal adenopathy need not just arise in the chest; it is also commonly seen in the lower neck. Because the deep cervical fascia encases the visceral space in a close-knit group, lesions arising in this region often obliterate the fat planes between thyroid, parathyroid, esophagus, and trachea, making determination of the origin of lesions more difficult.

Notes

Meningioma of the Sella

1. In less than one half of these patients the tumor can be dissected off the carotid artery without arterial injury or sacrifice. Because of the close approximation of cranial nerves III, IV, and especially VI to the cavernous carotid artery, extraocular motility is often compromised if the carotid artery is encased.

2. Approximately 10% of the time.

3. Adenoma, by far.

4. The orbital apex, the sphenoid sinus, the cavernous sinus, the optic nerves, and the chiasm.

Reference

Knosp E, Steiner E, Kitz K, Matula C: Pituitary adenomas with invasion of the cavernous sinus space: a magnetic resonance imaging classification compared with surgical findings, *Neurosurgery* 33:610-618, 1993.

Cross-Reference

Neuroradiology: THE REQUISITES, pp 302, 316-317, 323-324.

Comment

The article referenced above speaks to the imaging findings suggestive of cavernous sinus invasion with pituitary adenomas. In short, when there is tumor extension beyond the plane of the lateral aspects of the intra- and supracavernous carotid artery, there is cavernous sinus invasion in nearly all cases. When tumor does not cross the line from the center of the lumen of the carotid arteries, there is rarely if ever cavernous sinus invasion. If tumor crosses the center line between the carotids, the possibility of invasion is high. Hormonal levels are higher, tumor growth rates faster, CSF leak rates greater, and complete surgical extirpation rates lower when cavernous sinus invasion exists. Cavernous sinus invasion is the most frequent cause of incomplete surgical removal of pituitary adenomas.

Distinguishing between a pituitary adenoma and a diaphragma sellae meningioma is usually pretty simple when one can identify the pituitary gland separate from the mass. As these lesions grow, however, the normal gland may become obliterated. The presence of dural tails, bony reaction, carotid artery narrowing, and hyperdensity on unenhanced CT favors a meningioma. Intratumoral hemorrhage, sellar floor depression, and gross hormonal changes suggest pituitary adenomas.

Notes

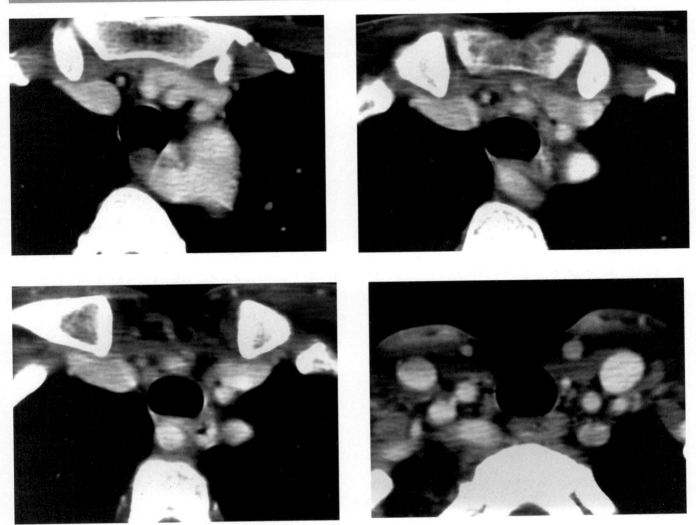

1. Describe the course (directionally) of this lesion.

2. From which embryologic vascular arch does the normal right proximal subclavian derive?

3. What is the most common anomaly of the aortic arch vessels?

4. What is the most common patient complaint with this anomaly?

Aberrant Right Subclavian Artery

1. The subclavian artery takes off from the distal aorta, passes behind the esophagus, and proceeds to the right axilla.

2. Arch number 4 on the right.

3. Aberrant right subclavian artery.

4. Nothing—most patients are asymptomatic. When they do complain, the symptoms are of difficulty swallowing (dysphagia lusoria).

Reference

Phillips WE II, Murtagh FR, Brenner J: Recognition of the aberrant right subclavian artery on cervical spine MR, *AJNR Am J Neuroradiol* 14:1405-1406, 1993.

Cross-Reference

Neuroradiology: THE REQUISITES, pp 435-436.

Comment

Coarctation of the aorta, tetralogy of Fallot, and interrupted aortic arches may coexist with an aberrant right subclavian artery. These disorders obviously overshadow any complaints caused by the subclavian artery impression on the esophagus. In association with a coarctation of the aorta, the aberrant subclavian artery may arise proximal or distal to the coarctation. Aberrancy of the right subclavian is a vascular lesion that used to be diagnosed on barium swallows—now it is more commonly seen as a serendipitous finding on a cross-sectional imaging study performed for other reasons. A prevalence rate of 0.5% to 2% has been reported.

Treatment of aberrant subclavian arteries (if required) usually consists of transposition of the vessel to the right common carotid artery. A cervical approach is favored over a median sternotomy. Aneurysms of the aberrant subclavian artery may occur and can be difficult to diagnose because of their unusual location. Rupture into the esophagus can be catastrophic.

Notes

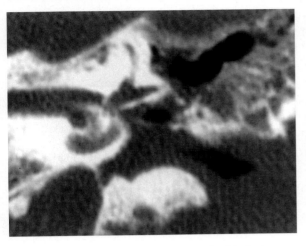 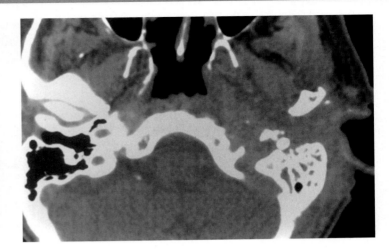

1. Describe the classic patient with this lesion.

2. What are the classic imaging features?

3. Common routes of spread?

4. Differential diagnosis?

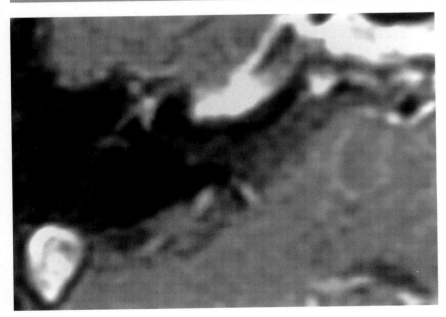

1. Which portions of the facial nerve may normally enhance?

2. What does the differential diagnosis of an enlarged, enhancing facial nerve in the temporal bone include?

3. What does the differential diagnosis of a nonenlarged, enhancing facial nerve in the temporal bone include?

4. What inflammatory lesions may cause facial nerve enhancement?

Malignant Otitis Externa

1. Elderly diabetic patient with external ear granulation who has recently had the ear irrigated.

2. External auditory canal thickening or mass, cortical bone erosion in the external auditory canal, and a soft tissue mass at the skull base.

3. To the skull base via the fissures of Santorini or sutures, to the nasopharynx via the eustachian tube, to the parapharyngeal space by direct spread, and superiorly through the tegmen tympani to the brain.

4. Nasopharyngeal carcinoma, skin cancer from the ear, and coalescent mastoiditis.

Reference

Grandis JR, Curtin HD, Yu VL: Necrotizing (malignant) external otitis: prospective comparison of CT and MR imaging in diagnosis and follow-up, *Radiology* 196:499-504, 1995.

Cross-Reference

Neuroradiology: THE REQUISITES, p 337.

Comment

On MRI, the granulation tissue of malignant otitis externa (MOE) classically is low on T1W and T2W scans, similar to a fungal infection, although MOE is caused by *Pseudomonas aeruginosa*. Patients may have cranial nerve symptoms owing to the involvement of the jugular foramen (and hence involvement of cranial nerves IX through XI) or the facial nerve in the temporal bone. Remember that resolution of findings of MOE on CT and MRI can be greatly delayed compared with clinical response. In fact, the erosive bony changes may persist indefinitely. Clinicians tend to rely on sedimentation rates and patient symptomatology to see if eradication of the *Pseudomonas* infection has occurred. If pushed for an imaging study to follow MOE, recommend a gallium scan, which reflects disease activity better than CT or MRI.

This CT shows opacification of the external ear, middle ear, and mastoid air cells with erosion of the superior wall of the external auditory canal. There is also obliteration of the fat planes at the base of the skull and parapharyngeal space with erosions of the anterior mastoid bone.

Notes

Enhancement of the Intralabyrinthine Portion of the Facial Nerve

1. The tympanic portion, geniculate ganglion, and intramastoid portion.

2. Schwannoma, hemangioma, perineural spread of tumors, sarcoidosis, and inflammatory/infectious lesions.

3. Usually an inflammatory lesion, but it may be a normal finding.

4. Infections from viral (HIV and herpetic), syphilitic, tuberculous, or Lyme disease or spread from otomastoiditis, with typical pathogens being *Pneumococcus, Streptococcus,* and *Haemophilus influenzae.* Noninfectious causes such as sarcoidosis may also cause similar findings.

Reference

Sartoretti-Schefer S, Wichmann W, Valvanis A: Idiopathic, herpetic, and HIV-associated facial nerve palsies: abnormal MR enhancement patterns, *AJNR Am J Neuroradiol* 15:479-485, 1994.

Cross-Reference

Neuroradiology: THE REQUISITES, p 353.

Comment

Idiopathic and herpetic causes account for over 85% of all unilateral peripheral facial nerve palsies. In this case there is enhancement of the facial nerve proximal to the geniculate ganglion. This is abnormal. One should never see facial nerve enhancement in the internal auditory canal or labyrinthine portion of the facial nerve. In fact, the distal intracanalicular segment is the most common site of abnormal facial nerve enhancement in patients with Bell's palsies. Occasionally, inner ear enhancement is seen with herpetic facial nerve palsy. Enhancement occurs at the distal intracanalicular labyrinthine junction (meatal foramen) because it is the narrowest intraosseous site of the fallopian canal. Therefore the nerve, when edematous, becomes ischemic, inflamed, and trapped. The blood-nerve barrier becomes disrupted—hence enhancement.

An entity to be aware of is Ramsay Hunt syndrome (herpes varicella zoster oticus). This disease is caused by herpetic infection involving the ear and is associated with a facial nerve palsy, vesicular lesions in the ear, and pain. The virus appears to be based in the geniculate ganglion. The eighth cranial nerve may also enhance in this syndrome.

James Ramsay Hunt was an American neurologist (1872-1937).

Notes

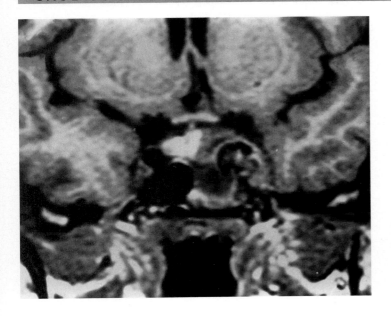
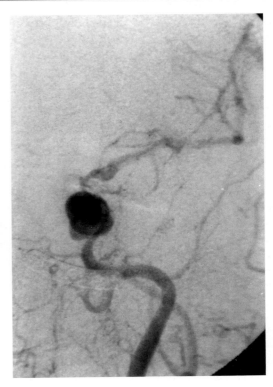

1. What are the causes of this lesion?
2. What is the best treatment?
3. What is the possible complication of this lesion?
4. What pulse sequence would be most helpful in this case?

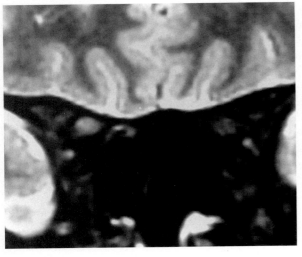
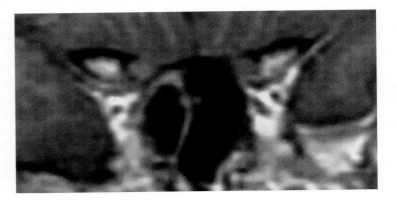

1. What are the salient findings on these scans?
2. What does the differential diagnosis of optic nerve or perioptic contrast enhancement include?
3. What percentage of patients with optic neuritis develop multiple sclerosis?
4. What are the characteristics of optic gliomas in adults as opposed to children?

Mycotic Aneurysm After Sphenoid Sinusitis

1. The aneurysm may occur spontaneously owing to virulent organisms growing into the cavernous sinus (especially fungus), or it may occur as an iatrogenic complication owing to sphenoid sinus surgery.

2. Endovascular occlusion when the infection is quiescent—otherwise, rupture can easily occur from the flimsy, infected wall of the aneurysm.

3. Cavernous carotid fistula, extravasation.

4. The raw data from the MRA.

Reference
Kennedy DW, Zinreich SJ, Hassab MJ: The internal carotid artery as it relates to endonasal sphenoethmoidectomy, *Am J Rhinol* 4:7-12, 1990.

Cross-Reference
Neuroradiology: THE REQUISITES, pp 180, 332.

Comment
Mycotic infections of the sinuses are curious beasts—they are rarely associated with air-fluid levels, even when acute. They have a far greater propensity for bony reaction and for vascular, skin, and orbital invasion than most bacterial infections. The vascular invasion is thought to be secondary to proteases expressed by the fungus that allow it to eat through vascular walls. This patient was treated endovascularly with occlusion of the ipsilateral internal carotid artery. Putting coils into an acutely inflamed, tenuous vessel only increases the risk of vascular rupture and is not a wise approach. "Trapping" the vessel or just occluding it proximally (and hoping it does not reconstitute via collaterals) seems more prudent acutely. Keep in mind that in 22% of patients there may be an area of dehiscence of the internal carotid artery wall along the posterior ethmoid or sphenoid sinus that predisposes one to injury at sinus surgery, to infectious aneurysms, and to sinonasal hemorrhage.

I am not a huge fan of MRA. A case like this, in which the variable signal intensity of fungus, hematoma, thrombus, slow flow, turbulence, and inspissated secretions may confound the study, bolsters the argument for having a low threshold to perform a conventional arteriogram.

Notes

Optic Neuritis

1. Abnormal bright signal intensity in the right optic nerve on the T2W scan (figure on left), and gadolinium enhancement of the nerve on the postcontrast, fat-saturated scan (figure on right).

2. Sarcoidosis, syphilis, tuberculosis, lymphoma, leukemia, CSF spread from melanoma, retinoblastoma, and other metastases; vasculitis; ischemic optic neuropathy; demyelinating disorders (multiple sclerosis); meningiomas; and optic nerve gliomas.

3. Fifty percent.

4. In children, optic gliomas are more commonly associated with neurofibromatosis and the benign pilocytic variety of astrocytomas. In adults, the optic gliomas are much more aggressive (anaplastic astrocytomas or glioblastoma multiforme) and have a more malignant course.

Reference
Millar WS, Tartaglino LM, Sergott RC, Friedman DP, Flanders AE: MR of malignant optic glioma of adulthood, *AJNR Am J Neuroradiol* 16:1673-1676, 1995.

Cross-Reference
Neuroradiology: THE REQUISITES, pp 290-291.

Comment
Optic neuritis can be easily imaged using fat-suppressed high resolution fast spin echo and/or fat-suppressed postgadolinium-enhanced MRI. This is an MRI diagnosis, not CT. A good quality 256×256 matrix fat-suppressed fast spin echo T2W scan is a beautiful way to demonstrate optic neuritis. Some programs are experimenting with a hybrid sequence that suppresses the CSF signal of the perioptic space in addition to the orbital fat to best demonstrate the optic nerve pathology. One-upmanship.

The entity is characterized by visual loss, pain on eye movement, and afferent pupillary defects. Although multiple sclerosis is a common cause, do not forget ischemic and vasculitic causes. With respect to optic gliomas, it is important to realize how aggressive these lesions can be in an adult as opposed to the namby-pamby optic gliomas seen with neurofibromatosis that have such a benign course. The former can spread like wildfire. Masses that can affect both the nerve and the sheath include optic glioma, lymphoma, pseudotumor, subarachnoid seeds, and melanoma.

Optic neuritis is the first manifestation of multiple sclerosis in 15% of patients and is seen in about 80% of patients with the disease. Devic syndrome (neuromyelitis optica) is optic neuritis (bilateral) with transverse myelitis—multiple sclerosis or acute disseminated encephalomyelitis may be the cause.

Notes

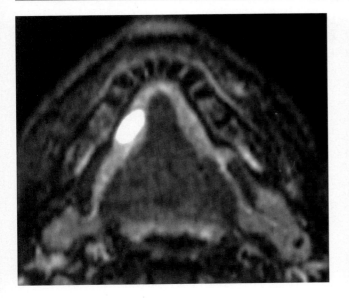 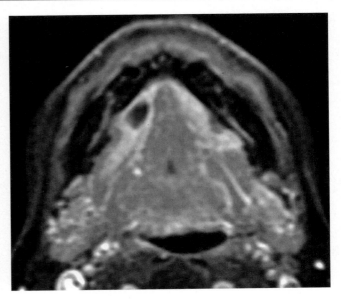

1. What does the differential diagnosis of a cytic lesion within the tongue include?

2. What is the cause of a ranula?

3. How does one distinguish a plunging ranula from a simple ranula?

4. What is the significance of distinguishing between a simple ranula and a plunging ranula?

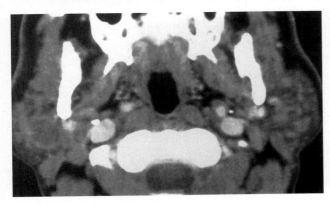 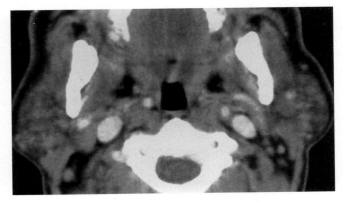

1. What tumor of the parotid gland has the highest rate of bilaterality?

2. When cysts are combined with nodules and are found bilaterally in the parotid glands, what diagnoses should be entertained?

3. Can the lymphoepithelial lesions associated with HIV positivity precede full-blown AIDS?

4. What does the differential diagnosis of a solitary cystic lesion in the parotid gland include?

Ranula

1. Dermoid cyst, epidermoid, lymphangioma, ranula, abscess, and thyroglossal duct cyst.

2. Ranulas occur owing to extravasation of mucous saliva from obstruction of the sublingual duct or minor salivary gland ducts in the floor of the mouth. Rarely obstruction of Wharton's duct may cause a ranula.

3. Simple ranulas stay in the floor of the mouth. Plunging ranulas perforate through or behind the mylohyoid muscle to enter the submandibular space.

4. Simple ranulas are treated via an intraoral approach. Plunging ranulas usually necessitate a cervical approach.

Reference

Morton RP, Bartley JR: Simple sublingual ranulas: pathogenesis and management, *J Otolaryngol* 24:253-254, 1995.

Cross-Reference

Neuroradiology: THE REQUISITES, pp 390-391.

Comment

There is now a debate regarding the pathogenesis of the ranula. Some believe that the lesion is due to either trauma to or infection of the sublingual duct and gland. This leads to extravasation of salivary secretory mucus into the sublingual tissue and encapsulation by connective tissue—hence the new term proposed, "mucus escape reaction." Others believe it is due to obstruction of the duct and that an epithelium-lined cyst develops (the classic ranula). Plunging ranulas often occur in the surgical bed of an incompletely removed simple ranula—scar formation from the intraoral surgery forces the expanding mass through the floor of the mouth into the submandibular space.

Ranulas often have relatively thick enhancing rims. Because the mouth is filled with potential pathogens, superinfection is quite common, so the lesion does not look like a pure wall-less cyst in most instances.

The Latin word for frog is *rana*. The ranula probably got its name from the similarity between a frog's neck and a patient's neck with a plunging ranula.

Notes

Lymphoepithelial Cysts and Nodules of the Parotid Gland Associated with HIV Positivity

1. Warthin's tumor (30%).

2. HIV-associated lymphoepithelial lesions, Sjögren's syndrome, and metastatic disease to the parotid glands.

3. Yes, very commonly.

4. Sialoceles, first branchial cleft cysts, mucous retention cysts, solitary lymphoepithelial cysts, pseudocysts, dermoid cysts, inclusion cysts, cystic neoplasms, and cystic hygromas.

Reference

Som PM, Brandwein MS, Silvers A: Nodal inclusion cysts of the parotid gland and parapharyngeal space: a discussion of lymphoepithelial, AIDS-related parotid, and branchial cysts, cystic Warthin's tumors, and cysts in Sjögren's syndrome, *Laryngoscope* 105:1122-1128, 1995.

Cross-Reference

Neuroradiology: THE REQUISITES, pp 416, 418-419.

Comment

Cysts and nodules in the parotid glands may be seen with HIV positivity, Sjögren's syndrome, Warthin's tumors, metastases (i.e., thyroid carcinoma), and sarcoidosis. The three types of lymphoid infiltrations of the parotid gland include (1) diffuse lymphocytic infiltration, (2) diffuse follicular lymphoid hyperplasia (as nodules), and (3) lymphoepithelial lesions (cysts and nodules) in the parotid gland. In patients with AIDS, adenovirus, mycobacterial infections, and fungi may infect the parotid gland. Lymphoma, Kaposi's sarcoma, or squamous cell carcinoma metastases may also be present because patients with AIDS do have an increased risk of these head and neck cancers.

Som refers to the lymphoepithelial cysts associated with HIV positivity as "AIDS-related parotid cysts (ARPCs)," but I do not like that term because many patients do not have AIDS when they have the cysts. The "cysts" are due to cystification within intraparotid nodes. Benign lymphoepithelial lesions (BLELs) can have cysts and nodules present as well. There is accompanying lymphocytic infiltration around the salivary ducts plus atrophy of the gland in BLELs of Sjögren's syndrome. ARPCs and BLELs have thin smooth walls and when solitary are therefore indistinguishable from first branchial cleft cysts. There is the potential for a BLEL of Sjögren's syndrome to undergo malignant degeneration into lymphoma. The clinical findings in the Sjögren's syndrome are (1) the sicca syndrome (dry eyes, dry mouth, dry skin) and (2) a connective tissue disorder (rheumatoid arthritis). The entity is seen most commonly in women (in a 9:1 ratio), usually in the fifth and sixth decades of life.

Notes

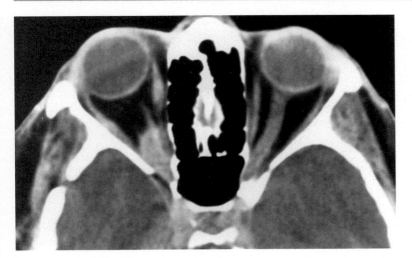

1. What is the classic CT description of an optic nerve meningioma?

2. What happens to the optic nerve sheath in pseudotumor cerebri?

3. What is arachnoid hyperplasia (gliomatosis), and with what is it associated?

4. Which affects vision earlier, an optic glioma or a meningioma?

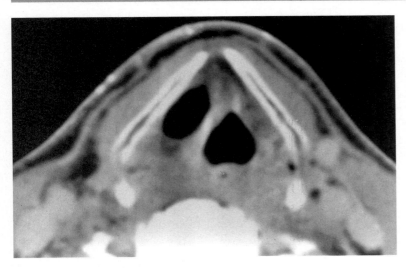

1. Who develop laryngoceles?

2. What are the types of laryngoceles, and how are they misnomers?

3. What maneuvers will distend a laryngocele?

4. Where do pharyngoceles (lateral pharyngeal pouches or diverticula) occur?

Optic Nerve Sheath Meningioma

1. Tram tracking (contrast enhancement) seen along the hypodense optic nerve.

2. It enlarges, and papilledema may occur.

3. Thickening of the optic nerve sheath meninges seen in association with optic nerve gliomas, especially in patients with neurofibromatosis.

4. Meningioma.

Reference

Ortiz O, Schochet SS, Kotzan JM, Kostick D: Meningioma of the optic nerve sheath, *AJNR Am J Neuroradiol* 17:901-906, 1996.

Cross-Reference

Neuroradiology: THE REQUISITES, pp 293-294.

Comment

Interestingly, 90% of intraorbital meningiomas arise from outside the orbit (planum, middle cranial fossa, sphenoid wing, dorsum sellae, tuberculum sellae, parasellar), and 4% of primary intraorbital meningiomas arise from arachnoid rests external to the optic nerve. In children, primary optic nerve sheath meningiomas are more common than secondary intraorbital extension (influenced in part by their association with neurofibromatosis). A classic history is a woman who develops vision loss during pregnancy—this is presumed to be due to growth of the tumor under the influence of estrogens and progesterones. Perioptic cysts may develop in patients with meningiomas and are not seen with optic gliomas.

One cautionary note: Tuberculum sellae and planum sphenoidale meningiomas may grow through the optic canal and present in a fashion similar to an optic nerve sheath meningioma. Not recognizing the intracranial component (which is exceedingly difficult on CT because these tumors may grow en plaque) can be disastrous for two reasons. There may be incomplete surgery that leaves residual tumor because the surgical plan discussed with the patient did not include a craniotomy. There may also be contralateral tumor growth from the planum or tuberculum that could affect both eyes. Monocular vision most people can live with. If both eyes are affected, early definitive intervention to afford some sight is critical. Remember that optic nerve meningiomas occur in children and in young and middle-aged adults—that would be many years without vision, many years paying off the malpractice suit. Look bilaterally!

Notes

Air-filled Laryngocele

1. Glass blowers, wind instrument players, chronic coughers or sneezers, and patients with laryngeal or pharyngeal masses.

2. Internal laryngoceles are contained by the thyrohyoid membrane; external laryngoceles extend out of the larynx, through the thyrohyoid membrane; and mixed laryngoceles have components in both spaces. By definition, all lesions communicate with the laryngeal saccule—therefore all external laryngoceles are truly mixed lesions. It's just that the dilated portion is outside the thyrohyoid membrane in external laryngoceles.

3. (Modified) Valsalva's maneuvers.

4. In the tonsillar fossa, paraglottic space, and piriform sinus region, and along the thyrohyoid membrane.

Reference

Glazer HS, Mauro MA, Aronberg DJ, Lee JK, Johnston DE, Sagel SS: Computed tomography of laryngoceles, *AJR Am J Roentgenol* 140:549-552, 1983.

Cross-Reference

Neuroradiology: THE REQUISITES, pp 396-397.

Comment

To me this is much ado about nothing—a little outpouching of the saccule of the laryngeal ventricle (sinus of Morgagni) that may be filled with air or fluid. The importance of the finding is to make sure there is not an obstructing mass in the ventricle. Laryngoceles are much more common in men than in women and in whites than in blacks. The mixed laryngocele is the most common kind. Bilateral laryngoceles occur in 32% of cases, and internal ones are twice as common as external ones.

Patients may complain of hoarseness or respiratory distress. Treatment of isolated internal laryngoceles may be through endoscopic laser therapy, whereas mixed laryngoceles necessitate an external incision.

Notes

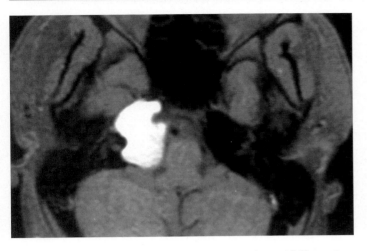 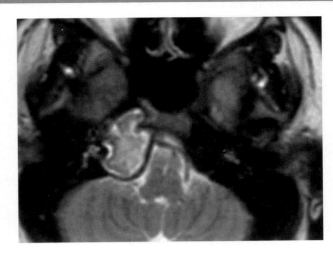

1. Can cholesterol granulomas occur in the middle ear?

2. What is the disadvantage of performing fast spin echo T2W scans in this setting?

3. Define Gradenigo's syndrome.

4. What critical structures are important to identify near any petrous apex mass?

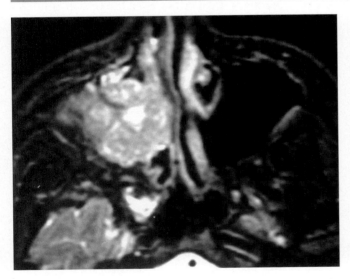 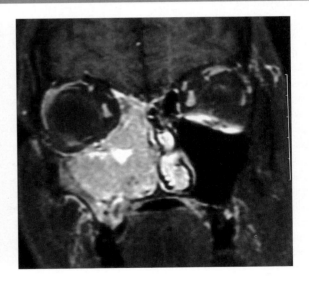

1. What are the imaging characteristics of an inverted papilloma?

2. Where are the most common locations of inverted papillomas?

3. What is the percentage of association with squamous cell carcinoma?

4. Can intracranial extent of the lesion occur?

Petrous Apex Mucocele

1. Absolutely. They are usually preceded by middle ear effusions and chronic otitis media.

2. Because petrous apex fat is bright on T1W scans, as well as on fast spin echo scanning, it is difficult to distinguish hemorrhagic lesions from normal bone marrow fat.

3. Otorrhea, fifth nerve facial pain, and sixth nerve palsy usually seen in patients who have petrous apicitis.

4. The internal carotid artery, the fifth cranial nerve, and the cavernous sinus. Additionally, the vertebral and basilar arteries may be affected by a lesion in this location.

Reference

Cheung SW, Broberg TG, Jackler RK: Petrous apex arachnoid cyst: radiographic confusion with primary cholesteatoma, *Am J Otol* 16:690-694, 1995.

Cross-Reference

Neuroradiology: THE REQUISITES, p 353.

Comment

Note that the T1W scan was performed with fat saturation, a nice technique to prevent mistakes caused by fat looking like pathology at the petrous apex. By all rights, this should be a cholesterol granuloma, but I could not convince the pathologist of that. Mucoceles of the petrous apex are not nearly as common as cholesterol granulomas. Schwannomas will enhance solidly, apicitis and mucoceles peripherally, and arachnoid cysts, cholesterol granulomas, and epidermoids not at all.

I guess the best reason to say that this is a petrous apex mucocele and not a cholesterol granuloma is that the lesion is not bright on T2W scans. Cholesterol granulomas are usually bright on both T1W and T2W scans, so maybe this lesion's intensity characteristics are due to inspissated protein, not blood products. I can buy that because intracellular methemoglobin (bright on T1W and dark like this on T2W scans) is the least commonly seen hemorrhagic by-product in head and neck radiology. I have seen a few cholesterol granulomas with mixed intensity on T2W scans. Bottom line: Petrous apex mucoceles and cholesterol granulomas are hard to distinguish when they are bright on T1W scans.

Notes

Inverted Papilloma

1. Intermediate signal intensity on T2W scanning, and solid, enhancing tissue. The lesion may have some calcification or residual bone fragments within it.

2. They most frequently arise from the lateral walls of the nasal cavity and nasal septum and from the walls of the maxillary antrum (in that order).

3. Roughly 12% to 15%.

4. Yes (same as with sinonasal polyposis).

Reference

Yousem DM, Fellows DW, Kennedy DW, Bolger WE, Kashima H, Zinreich SJ: Inverted papilloma: MR evaluation, *Radiology* 185:501-506, 1992.

Cross-Reference

Neuroradiology: THE REQUISITES, p 371.

Comment

I believe that it is impossible to distinguish between an inverted papilloma and a carcinoma. Both are intermediate in signal intensity on T2W scans, and both enhance solidly. It used to be that if you saw calcification in an intranasal polypoid mass, you would suggest a chondroid lesion, olfactory neuroblastoma, and inverted papilloma. Even this simple differential diagnosis has been discredited by some who believe the "calcification" that we have been seeing is really only destroyed bony septa or reactive native bone rather than true new bone formation within the inverted papilloma.

Inverted papillomas account for 4% of all nasal neoplasms and are bilateral in less than 5% of cases. The etiologic agent may be a human papillomavirus that affects men more than women. Recurrence rates are high, and the risk of a coexistent squamous cell carcinoma makes complete extirpation critical.

Som has noted that whereas the bones of the sinonasal cavity tend to remodel in response to a chronically expanding mass, those of the anterior and middle cranial fossa respond with osteolysis. Therefore one can see what looks like aggressive deossification in the cribriform plate and sphenoid wing regions even with benign masses. Bone loss in the walls of the sinonasal cavity, however, implies an aggressive lesion (though it may be inflammatory like some fungal infections).

Notes

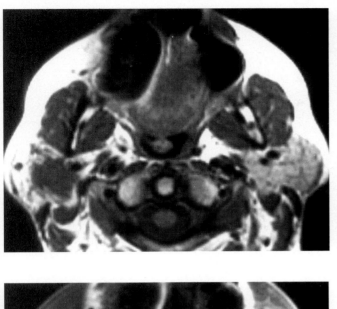
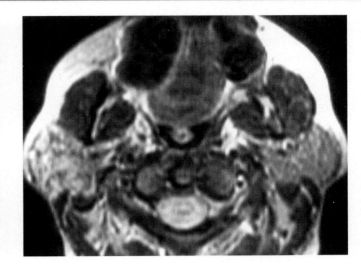
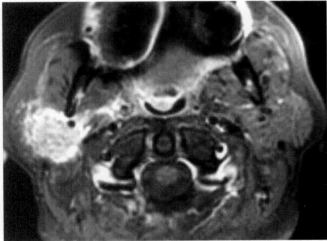

1. How reliable is the finding of irregular margins in predicting whether a parotid mass is malignant or benign?

2. How reliable is signal intensity in determining whether a parotid mass is benign or malignant?

3. What is the most common malignancy in the parotid gland?

4. What is the significance of describing whether a parotid mass is in the superficial or deep portion of the gland?

Mucoepidermoid Carcinoma of the Parotid Gland

1. Not very (approximately 60%).

2. Not very (approximately 73%).

3. Mucoepidermoid carcinoma.

4. The surgical approach may be different in a superficial lesion (in which the approach is usually with a skin incision around the ear) versus a deep lesion (in which the approach may be from the submandibular incision) versus a dumbbell superficial and deep lesion (in which the approach depends on the lesion's size but is usually via an incision around the ear).

Reference

Horowitz SW, Leonetti JP, Azar-Kia B, Fine M, Izquierdo R: CT and MR of temporal bone malignancies primary and secondary to parotid carcinoma, *AJNR Am J Neuroradiol* 15:755-762, 1994.

Cross-Reference

Neuroradiology: THE REQUISITES, pp 421-422.

Comment

Within the deep lobe of the parotid gland, the most common mass is a pleomorphic adenoma. The same holds true in the superficial lobe. One can tell whether the lesion is derived from the deep lobe of the parotid gland or the prestyloid parapharyngeal space minor salivary glands by the displacement of the parapharyngeal fat. Anteromedial displacement of the fat suggests that the lesion is arising from the deep lobe of the parotid gland. Encasement of the tumor by fat suggests a parapharyngeal origin. Sometimes this distinction is difficult to make, particularly with large masses.

In general, mucoepidermoid carcinomas may be bright or dark on T2W scans, varying with the grade of the tumor. Lower grade lesions are brighter than higher grade lesions, and the prognosis also correlates with T2W signal intensity because the higher grade lesions have a worse prognosis. The benign tumor of the parotid gland that classically appears in the tail of the gland is the Warthin's tumor.

Remember that skin (or external auditory canal) malignancies (basal cell and squamous cell carcinomas) may spread into or metastasize to the parotid gland. Therefore a cytologic aspirate that shows "malignant epidermoid cells" may be nondiagnostic because both squamous cell carcinoma and mucoepidermoid carcinoma may contain these cells. The prognosis for the former is vastly worse than that for the latter.

Notes

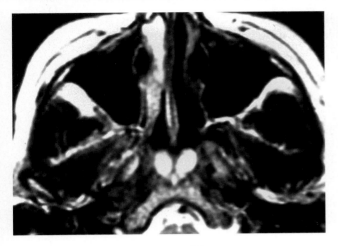
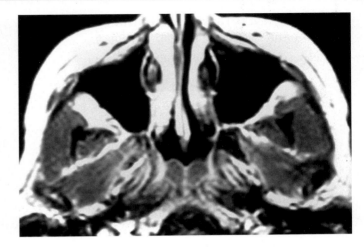

1. Why are these not Tornwaldt cysts?
2. What are obstructed with mucous retention cysts?
3. What structure demarcates the inferior margin of the nasopharynx posteriorly?
4. What structure demarcates the inferior margin of the oropharynx posteriorly?

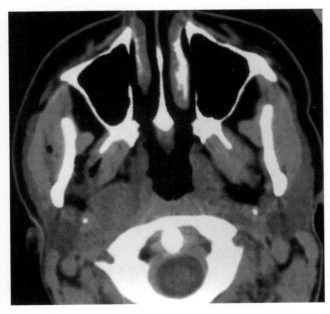

1. In what space is this mass?
2. If one cannot identify the styloid process (usually invisible on MRI), what can one use to determine whether a lesion is in the prestyloid parapharyngeal space or the carotid space?
3. From which branchial cleft does this cyst arise?
4. What study is critical for distinguishing a pleomorphic adenoma of the parapharyngeal space from a parapharyngeal space branchial cleft cyst?

Nasopharyngeal Mucous Retention Cysts

1. They are off midline and multiple.

2. Submucosal minor salivary glands or mucinous glands.

3. The hard palate–soft palate plane.

4. The pharyngoepiglottic folds.

Reference

Armengot M, Martinez-Sanjuan V, Martorell M, Basterra J: Retention cysts of the rhinopharynx: a case report, *Acta Otorhinolaryngol Belg* 50:199-201, 1996.

Cross-Reference

Neuroradiology: THE REQUISITES, pp 369-370.

Comment

It is very important to understand head and neck anatomy. As one runs down the posterior pharyngeal wall from the skull base to the esophagus, one passes from nasopharynx (skull base to hard palate–soft palate level) to oropharynx (hard palate–soft palate level to pharyngoepiglottic folds) to hypopharynx (pharyngoepiglottic folds to cricopharyngeus). The hard palate is actually part of the oral cavity, the soft palate part of the oropharynx, and the pharyngoepiglottic folds and postcricoid region part of the hypopharynx. Remember also that the tongue is separated into the base (oropharynx) and the oral tongue (oral cavity) and that the anteromedial margin of the piriform sinus (hypopharynx) is actually the lateral wall of the aryepiglottic fold (the supraglottic larynx). Confusing enough? Nonetheless, these boundaries are important to know because staging of lesions requires a knowledge of both the site of origin of the tumors and the extent of the lesion.

Mucous retention cysts can occur anywhere in the aerodigestive tract where there are mucin secreting cells or minor salivary gland rests. The nasopharynx and the walls of the eustachian tubes are not uncommon sites for these sorts of cysts. They are usually dark on T1W scans, unlike Tornwaldt cysts. The mucous retention cysts associated with the eustachian tubes may appear submucosal and may parallel the tensor and levator veli palatini muscles. They may have a nipple in the deep lateral recess and a protruding polypoid appearance extending into the airway.

Notes

Branchial Cleft Cyst (Ignore the Air from My Aspiration Procedure)

1. The prestyloid parapharyngeal space.

2. The styloid musculature (stylopharyngeus, stylohyoideus, styloglossus).

3. The second branchial cleft.

4. A contrast-enhanced scan.

Reference

Benson MT, Dalen K, Mancuso AA, Kerr HH, Cacciarelli AA, MaFee MF: Congenital anomalies of the branchial apparatus: embryology and pathologic anatomy, *Radiographics* 12:943-960, 1992.

Cross-Reference

Neuroradiology: THE REQUISITES, pp 336, 416, 429-431.

Comment

Second through fourth branchial cleft tissue makes up the cervical sinus of His, which obliterates in embryologic development. Second arch tissue is associated with the facial nerve, and therefore one should think of muscles of facial expression, hyoid tissue, middle ear incus and malleus, and stapedius muscles. Second pouch tissue develops into the palatine tonsil. The tract of the second branchial apparatus passes from the midportion of the sternocleidomastoid muscle, between the internal and external carotid arteries to the palatine tonsil. Four types of second branchial cleft cysts are recognized that follow the path from skin surface to tonsil. Type I cysts are posterior to the carotid bifurcation along the sternocleidomastoid muscles. Type II cysts are the most common and are closely apposed to the carotid bifurcation and the angle of the mandible. This case probably represents a Type III cyst, just deep to the pharynx in the parapharyngeal tissues. Type IV cysts appear submucosally along the pharyngeal wall.

In this case note that the lesion resides anterior and medial to the styloid process. Therefore one would not suggest other parapharyngeal lesions such as glomus tumors or vagal schwannomas. These lesions would lie behind the styloid process. Normally one performs a contrast-enhanced CT or, better yet, an MRI to evaluate this lesion. This study was performed for a CT-guided aspiration.

Notes

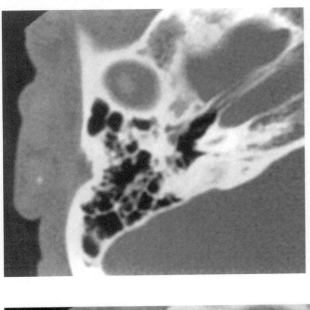
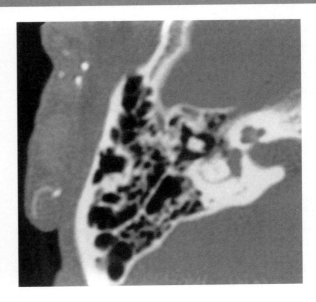
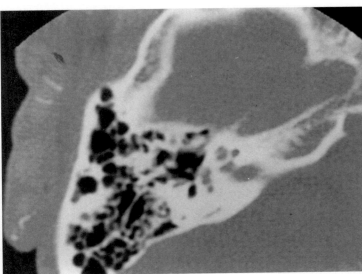
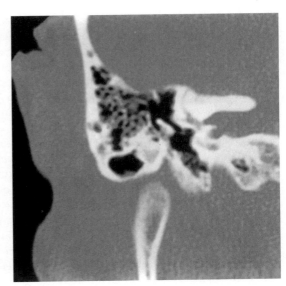

1. When describing congenital ear anomalies, what critical structures are important to identify and localize?

2. How often is aural atresia bilateral?

3. Which ossicles are usually affected with branchial arch I anomalies?

4. What is the cranial nerve most closely associated with branchial arch I structures?

Congenital External and Middle Ear Anomaly

1. The facial nerve, the carotid artery, the jugular vein, and areas of dehiscence in the bone. The degree of middle ear development is important because an adequately sized tympanic cavity and presence of ossicles are associated with a better outcome.

2. Thirty percent of the time.

3. The proximal malleus and proximal incus.

4. The mandibular nerve.

Reference

Lambert PR, Dodson EE: Congenital malformations of the external auditory canal, *Otolaryngol Clin North Am* 29:741-760, 1996.

Cross-Reference

Neuroradiology: THE REQUISITES, pp 336-337, 342.

Comment

With external auditory canal atresia, the malleus is usually more deformed than the incus, and the two are often fused, as in this case. The malleus may also be fused to the atretic bone of the external auditory canal laterally (seen here). The glenoid fossa and mandibular condyle may be poorly formed, and subluxation of the condyle out of the joint may be problematic, as was true in this patient.

First branchial anomalies should conjure up a vision of the third division of the fifth cranial nerve. The cartilage of the mesoderm, Meckel's cartilage, helps form the malleus, incus, and upper mandible. Muscles innervated by the mandibular nerve also come from the first arch mesoderm. The ectoderm of the first branchial apparatus forms the external auditory canal, and the endoderm forms the tympanic cavity, eustachian tube, and mastoid air cells. First branchial arch cysts are separated into two types: Arnot type I cysts are found in the lower parotid gland. Arnot type II cysts more commonly drain to the external auditory canal and are found in the deep lobe of the parotid, the upper periauricular region, or the anterior triangle of the neck.

The marked difficulty in hearing experienced by children with bilateral external auditory atresia is often corrected early on (age 5 to 6) to allow proper education of the child. With unilateral external auditory atresia, surgical correction (if performed at all) may be deferred until adolescence, at which time a single cosmetic surgery to reconstruct the auricle of the ear can be performed to achieve an adult ear configuration.

Treacher Collins syndrome, Crouzon's disease, Goldenhar's syndrome, Klippel-Feil disease, cleidocranial dysostosis, osteopetrosis, DiGeorge syndrome, and thalidomide toxicity are associated with external auditory canal stenoses or atresias.

Notes

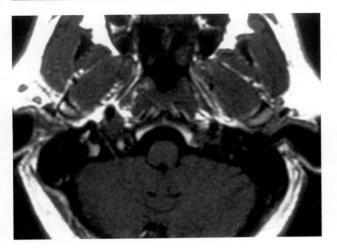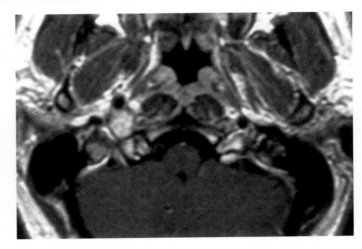

1. Why is this lesion not a glomus jugulare tumor?

2. If this lesion were a paraganglioma, what type would it be?

3. What else does the differential diagnosis of this lesion include?

4. What would be the leading diagnosis if the patient had a diminished gag reflex? Palatal palsy with an intact gag?

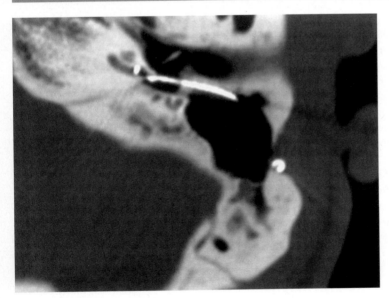

1. Is this the proper placement for cochlear implant leads?

2. How far in should a multichannel cochlear electrode go?

3. Through what anatomic structure is the cochlear implant inserted?

4. What are the contraindications to cochlear implantation?

Ninth Cranial Nerve Schwannoma

1. Because it does not grow into the jugular vein.

2. A glomus vagale paraganglioma.

3. Schwannoma, lymph node, pseudoaneurysm of the carotid artery, and other less common neurogenic tumors.

4. A ninth cranial nerve schwannoma for gag reflex. A tenth nerve schwannoma for palatal palsy.

Reference

Tay HL, Swanston AR, Lumley JS: Glossopharyngeal schwannoma presenting as gagging dysphagia, *Postgrad Med J* 70:207-209, 1994.

Cross-Reference

Neuroradiology: THE REQUISITES, pp 53, 311, 490.

Comment

Glossopharyngeal schwannomas are unusual tumors and are largely outweighed by glomus jugulare tumors in the differential diagnosis of a jugular foramen mass. The absence of growth into the jugular vein is the major factor in the argument against this tumor being a paraganglioma, although a glomus vagale, vagus schwannoma, and lymph node may appear similarly. Although most parapharyngeal schwannomas present because of their mass effect, a patient may experience subtle swallowing difficulties or globus sensations from these tumors when they are in the neck. Intracranial glossopharyngeal schwannomas may affect balance, gait, and hearing because of mass effect in the posterior fossa. Middle-aged adults or children with neurofibromatosis may present with ninth cranial nerve schwannomas. Whereas paragangliomas erode the jugular foramen and spine, most ninth cranial nerve schwannomas show a benign bony expansion of the pars nervosa (not vascularis) of the jugular foramen. Look for this difference in bony architecture to distinguish schwannomas from glomus tumors.

The glossopharyngeal nerve travels in the pars nervosa of the jugular foramen, which is anterior to the pars vascularis. Note that this lesion is anterior to the jugular vein but pushes the carotid artery, seen as a flow void, anteriorly. The vagus nerve and spinal accessory nerve travel with the jugular vein in the pars vascularis.

Notes

Cochlear Implantation into Round Window through Mastoidectomy (Canal Wall Up)

1. Not for a multichannel cochlear electrode, but possibly for a single channel cochlear electrode.

2. As far in as possible, but at least 2 to 3 cm (preferably at least into the middle cochlear turn).

3. The round window.

4. Congenital cochlear malformations, otospongiosis, and active infection.

Reference

Johnson MH, Hasenstab MS, Seicsnaydre MA, Williams GH: CT of postmeningitic deafness: observations and predictive value for cochlear implants in children, *AJNR Am J Neuroradiol* 16:103-109, 1995.

Cross-Reference

Neuroradiology: THE REQUISITES, p 351.

Comment

Childhood deafness can result from congenital deformities, meningitis (via spread from the meninges to the cochlear aqueduct), and idiopathic and iatrogenic (drug-induced) causes. Of those receiving cochlear implants, 44% are deaf as a complication of meningitis. These patients are at risk for developing obliterative cochlear stenosis that may be fibrous and/or ossific, hindering the placement of the cochlear implant. The basal turn is most commonly stenosed, and fibrous obliteration is more common than osseous obliteration—this accounts for most of the cases read as normal cochlea on CT but that fail at implant insertion. Ossification at the round window is another source of difficulty with electrode insertion but can be circumvented by localized drilling. After implantation, electrodes may migrate, programming of the device may be limited, and saturation of the limited neural tissue can occur. If problems arise, repeat cochlear implantation may be required, or the patient must suffer with limited function.

The bottom line with the 22 electrode cochlear implants is that the more electrodes you get deep into the cochlea, the better the hearing outcome. The likelihood of passing more than 10 electrodes into an ear with cochlear stenosis is only 30%.

I have seen seven cases of facial nerve stimulation by cochlear electrodes. This usually occurs secondary to dehiscence in the wall of the facial nerve canal along the basal turn of the cochlea.

Notes

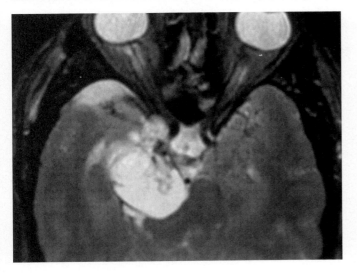 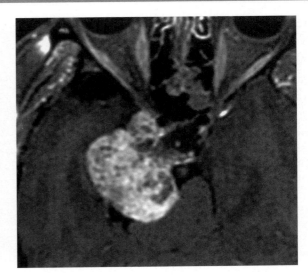

1. Do chordomas occur here?

2. With a calcified mass in the parasellar location, what is the most important diagnosis to consider?

3. What is the most common parasellar mass?

4. Do pituitary adenomas calcify?

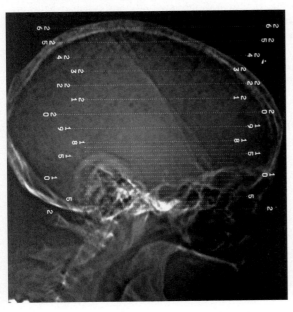 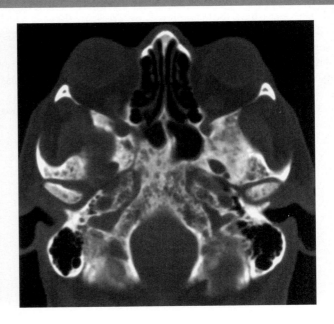

1. What neoplasms cause multiple lytic lesions in the skull base?

2. What nonneoplastic diagnoses can be considered with punctate lytic lesions of the skull?

3. What is the diagnosis if this lesion is not hot on bone scintigraphy?

4. How often are there no bone lesions identifiable in a patient with known multiple myeloma?

CASE 97

Parasellar Chondrosarcoma

1. Yes, parasellar chordomas are not uncommon.

2. An aneurysm.

3. A pituitary adenoma growing into the cavernous sinus.

4. Rarely, if ever.

Reference

Kunanandam V, Gooding MR: Parasellar chondrosarcoma: total excision improves prognosis, *Br J Neurosurg* 9:87-91, 1995.

Cross-Reference

Neuroradiology: THE REQUISITES, pp 326-330.

Comment

Chondrosarcomas account for 6% of the neoplasms of the skull base, but they tend to favor the sphenooccipital and petroccipital synchondroses along the clivus. From there they may grow into the parasellar region. They are fairly bright on T2W scans—but then again, so are chordomas, which are the main players in the differential diagnosis of skull base masses. Chondrosarcomas are a little more variable in their location than chordomas—people get more riled up with a petrous apex or cavernous sinus chordoma than with a chondrosarcoma. Patients less than 30 years old are affected most commonly.

Chondrosarcomas have been reported to arise in the meninges or the falx. Recurrence is a problem, but in general they are low grade lesions. The heterogeneous nature of this lesion and its marked hyperintensity on the T2W scan (figure on left), coupled with the absence of a dural tail, factor against this particular lesion being a meningioma. I would still put a meningioma high on my differential list because meningiomas occur so much more commonly than chondrosarcomas, but you could be a superstar by making the "zebra call." (Naaay?)

Notes

CASE 98

Multiple Myeloma of Skull Base

1. Metastases and multiple myeloma.

2. Mastocytosis, hyperparathyroidism, Langerhans cell histiocytosis, and osteoporosis circumscripta of Paget's disease.

3. Multiple myeloma.

4. Thirty percent of the time.

Reference

Avrahami E, Tadmor R, Kaplinsky N: The role of T2-weighted gradient echo in MRI demonstration of spinal multiple myeloma, *Spine* 18:1812-1815, 1993.

Cross-Reference

Neuroradiology: THE REQUISITES, p 495.

Comment

Gradient echo scans appear to be one of the most sensitive MRI series for the detection of multiple myeloma lesions, more so even than CT. The punched-out lesions here, though in an unusual site for multiple myeloma, are characteristic of the disorder elsewhere in the skeleton. The mean age for diagnosis of multiple myeloma is 66 years. The most common sites involved with myeloma are the spine (49%), skull (35%), pelvis (34%), and ribs (33%). In the head and neck, the mandible is most frequently affected. One of the disease's manifestations is osteopenia with or without vertebral body collapse. Scintigraphy is usually negative.

The diagnosis of multiple myeloma is made more frequently by reviewing the scout topogram (provided in this case) than the axial scans, especially with lesions at the vertex.

Notes

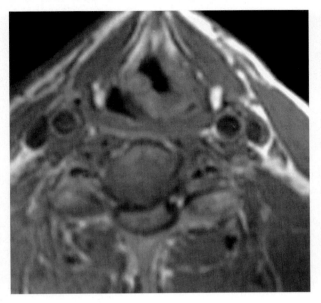 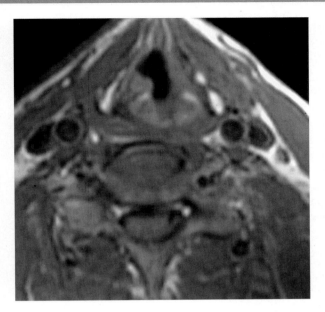

1. What should be the scanning range in the evaluation of left-sided and right-sided vocal cord paralysis?

2. What are the imaging findings of recurrent laryngeal nerve paralysis versus those of superior laryngeal nerve paralysis?

3. In what percentage of patients is a vocal cord paralysis caused by a neoplasm?

4. Name other causes of vocal cord paralysis.

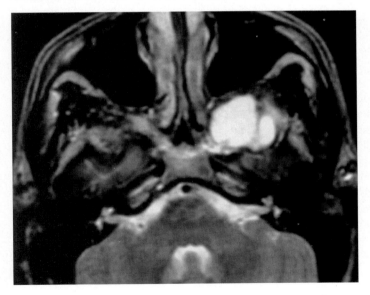 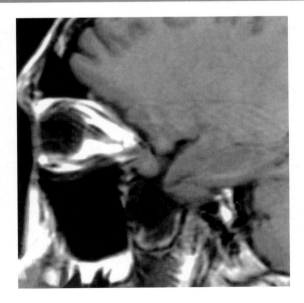

1. Into what space does this lesion appear to protrude?

2. What are common causes of meningoceles affecting the tegmen tympani?

3. How often is the jugular bulb congenitally dehiscent?

4. How often is the cribriform plate macroscopically dehiscent?

Right-sided Vocal Cord Paralysis

1. When scanning on the left side one should cover from the medulla through the skull base inferiorly to the middle mediastinum midheart level. When scanning on the right side one should cover from the medulla through the skull base to below the right subclavian artery.

2. Recurrent laryngeal nerve paralysis: (1) dilatation or enlargement of the vallecula, piriform sinus, and laryngeal ventricle; (2) adduction of the vocal cord, rotation of the cricoarytenoid joint more medially, and medial orientation of the false vocal cord. (3) The cord may thin when the process is chronic. With a superior laryngeal nerve paralysis one usually sees nothing on imaging.

3. Approximately 30% to 45%. (Neoplasm is the most common cause; lung is the most common primary site.)

4. From most to least common—postoperative (especially parathyroid and thyroid surgery)/iatrogenic, idiopathic, goitrous, inflammatory, traumatic (especially after intubation), and central (intracerebral) causes.

Reference
Terris DJ, Arnstein DP, Nguyen HH: Contemporary evaluation of unilateral vocal cord paralysis, *Otolaryngol Head Neck Surg* 107:84-90, 1992.

Cross-Reference
Neuroradiology: THE REQUISITES, pp 401-402.

Comment
The ratio of unilateral to bilateral vocal cord paralysis is approximately 3:1. There is a slight preference for the left vocal cord, possibly because of the more inferior location of the recurrent laryngeal nerve, exposing it to more lung pathology. The left nerve passes under the aortic arch; the right nerve passes under the right subclavian artery. The yield from imaging or clinical evaluation of vocal cord paralysis is reported to be about 75%, which seems a bit high based on my experience. The chest x-ray proves to be one of the most valuable imaging studies in this clinical scenario. MRI should probably follow if no lesion is discovered on plain film, with attention to the chest and specialized motion correction procedures applied. The muscle supplied by the superior laryngeal nerve (a branch of the vagus) is the cricothyroid muscle. If both superior laryngeal and recurrent laryngeal nerves are affected the cord is intermediate in location (completely adducted). If just the recurrent laryngeal nerve is affected the cord is paramedian.

Notes

Meningocele of Middle Cranial Fossa

1. It extends into the pterygopalatine fossa and masticator space (infratemporal fossa).

2. Congenital traumatic, and postoperative causes. They also occur secondary to cholesteatomas with tegmen dehiscence.

3. Approximately 8% of the time.

4. Three percent of the time.

Reference
Raftopoulos C, David P, Allard S, Ickx B, Baleriaux D: Endoscopic treatment of an oral cephalocele, *J Neurosurg* 81:308-312, 1994.

Cross-Reference
Neuroradiology: THE REQUISITES, pp 273-274.

Comment
David Kennedy has taught me to use the term cephaloceles at our institution (and has asked me to pronounce it with a *k* sound). I am not sure if this is because I have been proven to be so bad at predicting whether there is brain, meninges, or both in the defect that is identified on imaging. In this case it looks like only the meninges and CSF are herniating through the skull defect. Note also that the lesion extends just posterior to the maxillary antrum on the sagittal scan and that therefore the pterygopalatine fossa is involved.

Most cephaloceles arise from the occipital bone in association with Arnold-Chiari malformations (type III) or along the cribriform plate in association with trauma or postoperative defects. CT, to demonstrate the bony dehiscence, and MRI, to demonstrate the contents of the cephalocele, should be used in concert to best characterize the lesion for the neurosurgeon or endoscopic sinus surgeon who repairs these. Three-dimensional CT is particularly elegant in giving the surgeon an idea of the location and extent of the hole that must be patched. With temporal or sphenoid bone cephaloceles, the site of dehiscence may be at the sphenopetrosal suture or the foramen lacerum. These cephaloceles present later because the defect is not visible, and often the presenting symptom is seizure or CSF leak. Heterotopic brain tissue may also be seen in either the pterygopalatine fossa or the orbit.

Notes

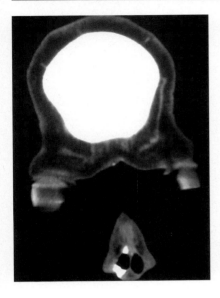
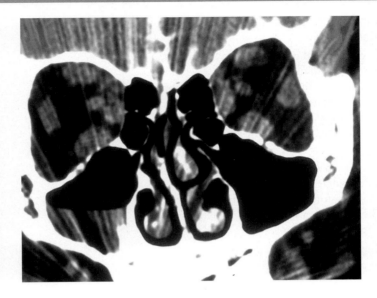

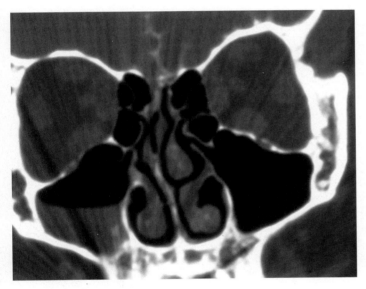

1. How is the study shown performed?

2. Can CSF leaks be repaired from below?

3. What are some of the causes of CSF leaks in this location?

4. What substance is typically tested for to determine whether fluid in the sinuses comes from sinonasal secretions or the CSF?

Cerebrospinal Fluid Leak along Cribriform Plate

1. Nonionic contrast material is instilled via a lumbar puncture. The patient is manipulated into a head-down position and rotated to place the contrast material into the dependent side where the leakage is suspected. Thin-section CT is performed in the appropriate (hyperextended supine) position, usually in the coronal plane.

2. Yes, with success rates of 75% to 85%. In fact, endoscopic repairs with fat or myocutaneous grafts, free tissue composite grafts of turbinate bone, submucosal tissue and mucosa, and mucosal grafting (held together with fibrin "glue") have become big business for the functional endoscopic sinus surgeons.

3. Trauma; postoperative, iatrogenic, idiopathic, and congenital causes; pseudotumor cerebri; and masses.

4. ß-2-Transferrin.

Reference

Lloyd MN, Kimber PM, Burrows EH: Post-traumatic cerebrospinal fluid rhinorrhea: modern high-definition computed tomography is all that is required for the effective demonstration of the site of leakage, *Clin Radiol* 49:100-103, 1994.

Cross-Reference

Neuroradiology: THE REQUISITES, p 20.

Comment

Despite the title of the article cited above, most CSF leaks caused by dural tears are best assessed with a combination of studies. Nuclear medicine studies in which indium–diethylenetriamine pentaacetic acid is injected intrathecally are highly accurate for detecting leaks when active flow is present, even at a slow rate. Pledgets are placed in the nose, and counts are recorded comparing right and left sides, superior and inferior quadrants. However, the anatomic definition afforded by CT makes a postcisternogram CT study more useful to the clinician. If there is rapid, active CSF leakage, the CT may show the contrast dye in the sinonasal cavity at the site of intracranial dehiscence. The endoscopic treatment of this complication can best be guided by the CT because the bony dehiscence can usually be seen and the landmarks to the site delimited. If, however, the possibility of brain herniating through the dehiscent area is a question, MRI is of value. It may also distinguish postoperative scar tissue or inflammation from meninges, CSF, and brain. Despite the relative contributions of imaging, direct endoscopic visualization of intrathecally instilled fluorescein leaking from the cribriform plate is the most reliable test in a skilled endoscopist's hands.

Notes

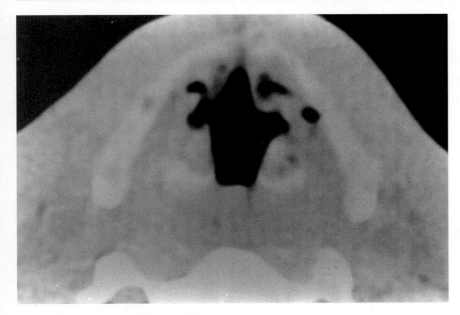

1. What is evident on these films?

2. In a patient with laryngeal trauma, what is the most likely source of extraluminal air?

3. What is the mechanism of injury in most cases of laryngeal trauma?

4. What is the ratio of incidence of mucosal tears to laryngeal fractures in patients with laryngeal trauma?

CASE 103

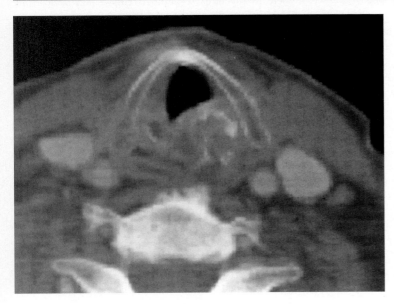

1. Is this lesion mucosal or submucosal in origin?

2. Are these lesions usually bright or dark on MRI?

3. Can one have benign chondroid tumors of the larynx?

4. Are chondrosarcomas of the larynx aggressive lesions?

Laryngeal Mucosal Tear

1. Gas in the paraglottic soft tissues.

2. Most likely a mucosal tear from the false cord level.

3. Crush injury of the thyroid cartilage during an auto accident.

4. One to one.

Reference

Snow JB Jr: Diagnosis and therapy for acute laryngeal and tracheal trauma, *Otolaryngol Clin North Am* 17:101-106, 1984.

Cross-Reference

Neuroradiology: THE REQUISITES, pp 395-403.

Comment

Laryngeal trauma, usually from a blunt injury to the neck during a high-speed collision, is a common cause of laryngotracheal stenosis. The longer one's neck the more likely the trauma will affect the supraglottic region rather than subglottic or tracheal zones. When extraluminal air is seen, laryngeal, pharyngeal, and esophageal mucosal tears and/or tracking of air from a pneumomediastinum must be considered. Early repairs of mucosal tears, especially those with cartilage exposed, produce the best long-term results. Problems involving infection of the cartilage can lead to long-term difficulties in maintaining airway patency.

The differential diagnosis in this case includes a gas-forming organism infection and small irregular laryngoceles. Because mucosal tears do not occur spontaneously, the history of vehicular trauma with the obliteration of the subcutaneous fat in this patient's neck (indicative of edema) makes this a simple case. The patient is usually very tender over the trauma site, and crepitus may be palpated from the escaped air. Ecchymoses of the mucosa near the tear are seen at endoscopy.

Notes

Chondrosarcoma of the Larynx

1. Submucosal.

2. Bright except for the densely calcified areas.

3. Yes.

4. Not at all.

Reference

Froberg MK, Meschter SC, Brown RE, Garbes AD: Cartilaginous tumors of the larynx: a report of two cases with definitive diagnosis by fine needle aspiration and computed tomography, *Acta Cytol* 40:761-764, 1996.

Cross-Reference

Neuroradiology: THE REQUISITES, pp 329-330, 398-403.

Comment

The skinny on chondrosarcomas of the larynx is that they are slow-growing nonaggressive malignancies that can be resected without a generous cuff of normal tissue (unlike squamous cell carcinomas). Therefore the surgeon is more willing to perform a partial laryngeal (voice-sparing) operation without the same worry about clean margins. These are not killer lesions. Sarcomas account for less than 1% of all laryngeal tumors, and chondrosarcomas have an affinity for the cricoid cartilage. They expand the cartilage rather than destroy it like squamous cell carcinomas do. Another sarcoma that affects the larynx is malignant fibrous histiocytoma.

Elsewhere in the body, chondrosarcomas may arise from preexisting lesions such as enchondromas or osteochondromas. This is less commonly seen in the head and neck unless the patient has a multiple enchondromas syndrome. Maffucci's (Angelo Maffucci, Italian surgeon, 1845-1903) syndrome and Ollier's (Léopold Louis Xavier Edouard Ollier, French surgeon, 1830-1900) disease are associated with multiple enchondromas, but usually of the extremities.

Notes

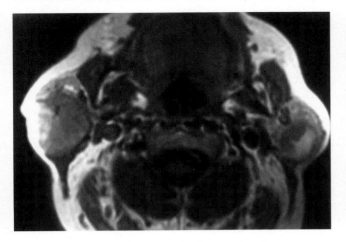
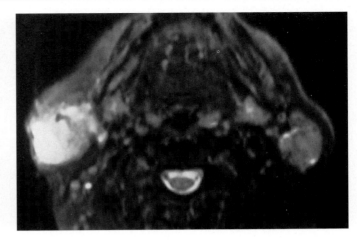

1. Describe the T staging of salivary gland tumors.

2. Distinguish between the ratio of benign to malignant salivary gland lesions in adults versus the same ratio in children.

3. What is the second most common benign tumor of the parotid gland in an adult?

4. Can Warthin's tumors occur in periparotid lymph nodes?

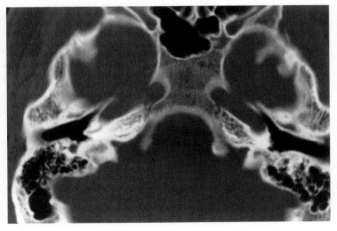
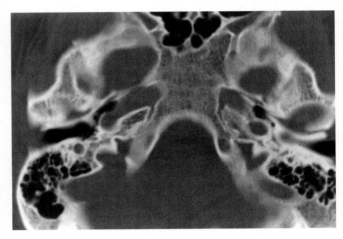

1. What structure is enlarged in this patient's right temporal bone?

2. What nerves arise from the facial nerve in its intramastoid portion?

3. What muscles are supplied by the facial nerve?

4. How often do patients with seventh cranial nerve schwannomas present with facial nerve palsies?

CASE 104

Warthin's Tumors of the Parotid Gland

1. T1—tumor 2 cm or less in greatest dimension; T2—tumor greater than 2 cm but less than or equal to 4 cm in greatest dimension; T3—tumor greater than 4 cm but less than or equal to 6 cm in greatest dimension; and T4—tumor greater than 6 cm in greatest dimension. There is a subdivision into A (no local extension) and B (local extension into the skin, soft tissue, bone, or nerves) types.

2. Whereas 1 in 5 tumors are malignant in the adult, 1 in 3 are malignant in children.

3. Warthin's tumor.

4. Yes, because they may arise within heterotopic salivary gland tissue within lymph nodes of the parotid or peri-parotid region.

Reference

Minami M, Tanioka H, Oyama K, Itai Y, Eguchi M, Yoshikawa K, Murakami T, Sasaki Y: Warthin tumor of the parotid gland: MR-pathologic correlation, *AJNR Am J Neuroradiol* 14:209-214, 1993.

Cross-Reference

Neuroradiology: THE REQUISITES, p 420.

Comment

Warthin's tumors violate the adage about T2W images that says what's bright is right in the parotid gland. In this case, the tumors are usually intermediate and inhomogeneous in signal intensity on T2W scans, yet the tumor is benign. The other names for this tumor—papillary cystadenoma lymphomatosum, adenolymphoma, lymphomatous adenoma, and cystadenolymphoma—speak to its varied histologic contents, which have countervailing T2W intensities. A predilection for the tail of the parotid gland is noted with Warthin's tumors.

Recent data suggest that smoking is a risk factor for the development of Warthin's tumors because patients with Warthin's tumors are 4 times more likely to smoke than age-matched controls or patients with pleomorphic adenomas of the parotid glands. Number of packs per day and years smoking appear to correlate with the risk of developing Warthin's tumors. Men are affected more often than women, at a rate of 5:1, which is in contrast to pleomorphic adenomas.

Warthin's tumors have thin capsules, as well as intratumoral septations and hemorrhage on occasion. Hyperproteinaceous debris, lymphoid follicles, reactive lymphocytes, and cholesterol crystals may be present. Cystic areas are present in 30% of cases.

Notes

CASE 105

Right Seventh Cranial Nerve Schwannoma

1. The descending portion of the right facial nerve canal.

2. The chorda tympani and the nerve to the stapedius muscle.

3. The muscles of facial expression, the platysma, the stylohyoid muscle, the posterior belly of the digastric muscle, and the stapedius muscle.

4. Twenty-five percent to 50% of the time.

Reference

Chen JM, Moll C, Wichmann W, Kurrer MO, Fisch U: Magnetic resonance imaging and intraoperative frozen sections in intratemporal facial schwannomas, *Am J Otol* 16: 68-74, 1995.

Cross-Reference

Neuroradiology: THE REQUISITES, p 347.

Comment

The facial nerve schwannoma may arise in the cerebellopontine angle cistern, the internal auditory canal, the temporal bone, the stylomastoid foramen, the parotid gland, or the face. At the geniculate ganglion, the schwannoma may locally expand the bone, creating a "crescent sign." With extracranial schwannomas, the facial nerve is less frequently involved than the vagus, sympathetic plexus, cervical plexus, or trigeminal nerves. Signal intensity on T2W scans varies according to the ratio of Antoni A and B tissue, the latter being bright and the former dark on long TR scans. Dynamic scanning showing persistent uptake in the mass without an early dip in enhancement distinguishes schwannomas from paragangliomas. On angiography they are much less vascular than glomus tumors. Interestingly enough, gadolinium-enhanced MRI may be even more helpful in planning the surgical approach and in defining the extent of tumor involvement relative to the facial nerve than intraoperative frozen sections, which frequently overestimate tumor extent.

Seventh nerve palsies can lead to weakness in the bottom eyelid and deficits in upper eyelid closure, but ptosis is a third nerve symptom. With a third nerve palsy the eye can still be shut tightly because of intact seventh nerve fibers. You may see a gold weight placed in the eyelid of a person with a seventh nerve palsy to assist in shutting the eye.

Notes

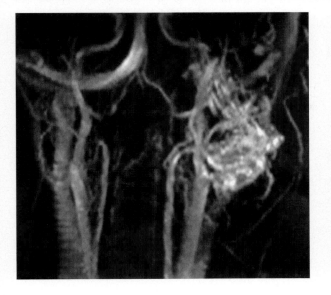
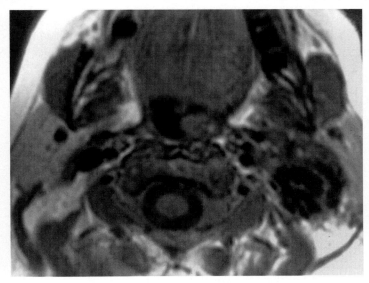
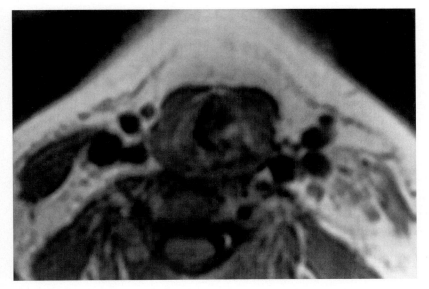

1. Based on the imaging findings provided, which cranial nerves appear to show damage?

2. Where do the findings above suggest the pathology resides?

3. What is the significance of the nodose ganglion?

4. What is the significance of pharyngeal abnormalities in a patient who has a vocal cord paralysis?

Neck Arteriovenous Malformation

1. Cranial nerve X (palatal palsy with uvula deviated to left in figure in upper right, vocal cord paralysis in figure in lower left) and cranial nerve XI (sternocleidomastoid atrophy).

2. In the medulla, the jugular foramen, or the proximal carotid sheath.

3. It is thought to be the origin of the glomus vagale tumor, and it is located in the carotid space at the nasopharyngeal level.

4. This suggests that the lesion is above the level of the hyoid bone because the ninth cranial nerve, as well as the pharyngeal plexus of the tenth cranial nerve, is also affected.

Reference

Baker LL, Dillon WP, Hieshima GB, Dowd CF, Frieden IJ: Hemangiomas and vascular malformations of the head and neck: MR characterization, *AJNR Am J Neuroradiol* 14:307-314, 1993.

Cross-Reference

Neuroradiology: THE REQUISITES, pp 144-145, 296, 326-327.

Comment

This is a wonderful case showing the effects of cranial nerve injury from a vascular malformation. Simply beautiful. Although head and neck vascular malformations are present at birth, they do not seem to produce symptoms until the end of the first or beginning of the second decade of life. Venous malformations and hemangiomas of the neck may be detected at birth as a result of skin discoloration or a soft tissue mass. Venous malformations do not involute, whereas childhood hemangiomas do. The vascular malformations respond to the vagaries of endocrinologic changes (adolescence, pregnancy, hormonal pharmaceuticals) and superimposed infection or to changes in vascular volume. Skeletal abnormalities may be seen in up to 35% of patients with head and neck vascular malformations owing to the effects of body growth, a steal phenomenon, remodeling from mass effect, or growth into the bone.

There really is no such thing as a ninth nerve palsy because it is predominantly a sensory nerve with motor innervation only to the stylopharyngeus muscle. A diminished gag reflex occurs owing to the absent sensory input, not owing to palatal paralysis. The palatal musculature is innervated by the vagus nerve. Sensation of the palate is best tested with gentle and painful stimuli to elicit ninth nerve signs of pathology. Pain in the region of the external auditory canal may be seen with both ninth and tenth nerve lesions.

Notes

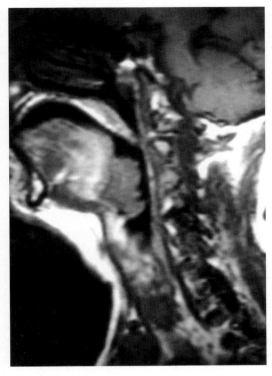

1. In what part of the aerodigestive tree is the base of the tongue?

2. Why are base of tongue cancers associated with a worse prognosis than oral tongue cancers?

3. What is the significance of preepiglottic fat invasion with oropharyngeal tumors, and is it invaded here?

4. What is the significance of extension of the mass across the midline of the base of the tongue?

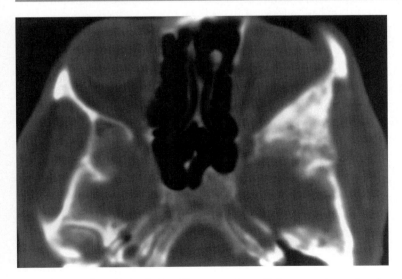

1. What is the clinical significance of medial versus lateral sphenoid wing meningiomas?

2. Why is MRI superior to CT for evaluating this lesion?

3. What does the differential diagnosis of this lesion include?

4. Is osteolysis more commonly seen than hyperostosis in association with meningiomas?

Base of Tongue Cancer

1. The oropharynx.

2. There is early bilateral lymph node drainage producing metastatic cervical adenopathy.

3. It makes the tumor a T4 cancer, means that the patient requires a supraglottic laryngectomy at least, and is associated with an even higher rate of nodal metastases. No, the preepiglottic fat is not invaded in this patient, as evidenced by the clean bright fat stripe below the tumor anteroinferior to the epiglottis.

4. A total glossectomy—which leaves the patient with a much worse quality of life than a hemiglossectomy, after which one can still eat and speak fairly intelligibly—will probably be required.

Reference

Loevner LA, Yousem DM, Montone KT, Weber R, Chalian AA, Weinstein GS: Can radiologists accurately predict preepiglottic space invasion with MR imaging? *AJR Am J Roentgenol* 169:1681-1688, 1997.

Cross-Reference

Neuroradiology: THE REQUISITES, p 392.

Comment

Sagittal and axial T1W scans are the best pulse sequences to view when trying to evaluate the preepiglottic fat for invasion. Invasion may occur with base of tongue, vallecular, or supraglottic cancers and means that the patient will require either a supraglottic or total laryngectomy. MRI is very sensitive in the detection of tumor spread into this fat-filled region, but edema and partial volume effects can hurt its specificity. Paraglottic extension may also change the extent of surgery, often forcing a supracricoid or total laryngectomy. Equally as important is the presence of bilateral tongue base invasion. One can live fairly well with a hemiglossectomy, although speech is affected and less intelligible. However, with a total glossectomy, one can no longer form a bolus with the back of the tongue, and swallowing becomes birdlike. Many patients ultimately require permanent gastrostomy tubes. The decision to live a mute life with a tracheostomy for breathing (because of a total laryngectomy) and a feeding gastrostomy (because of a total glossectomy) is a very tough one to make, and many patients opt out of surgery. Unfortunately, for advanced disease necessitating those operations, radiation therapy has low success rates. Ultimately, it becomes a quality of life versus quantity of life issue.

Many surgeons believe that vallecular mucosa involvement forces them to remove a cuff of epiglottis and epiglottic fat to get clean margins. The implications are not nearly as dire as those of true preepiglottic fat invasion, however, because of nodal considerations.

Notes

Intraosseous Meningioma

1. The medial ones are much harder to resect (because of proximity to the cavernous sinus) and have a higher rate of cranial nerve involvement.

2. Because the MRI is more likely to be able to detect the small dural component of the intraosseous meningioma.

3. Metastatic bone disease, fibrous dysplasia, Paget's disease, and intraosseous meningioma.

4. Yes.

Reference

Terstagge K, Schorner W, Henkes H, Heye N, Hosten N, Lanksch WR: Hyperostosis in meningiomas: MR findings in patients with recurrent meningioma of the sphenoid wings, *AJNR Am J Neuroradiol* 15:555-560, 1994.

Cross-Reference

Neuroradiology: THE REQUISITES, p 70.

Comment

Hyperostosis of bone can be seen in about one third of all meningiomas that are located along the anterior skull base and has been reported in 4.5% to 45% of cases—highly variable. It seems that the variability of hyperostosis depends on the site of origin of the meningioma—rare over the convexities, not unusual at the skull base (as high as 90% along the sphenoid wing). Is it tumor in the bone or just reactive osteoblasts or hypervascularity that does it? The evidence favors a component of tumoral infiltration of the bone. Contrast enhancement of the bone on MRI scanning is indicative of neoplastic infiltration. In fact, the whole idea of intraosseous meningiomas has been called into question because there is almost always a piece of dura that enhances adjacent to the bone.

Osteoblastic metastases are most commonly seen with breast cancer and prostate cancer. Lung, bladder, and gastrointestinal primary lesions may cause osteosclerotic metastases, as can lymphoma. Chronic osteomyelitis, syphilis, and primary bone sarcomas can cause similar appearances.

Notes

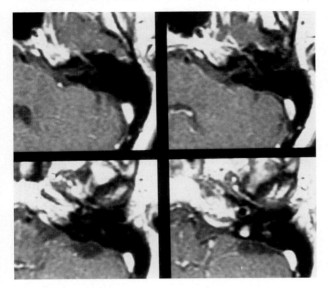

1. How often does the facial nerve in asymptomatic individuals enhance on MRI?

2. How often is that enhancement asymmetric from side-to-side?

3. What is the most common symptom associated with intratemporal facial nerve schwannomas?

4. What cranial nerve is affected most commonly in sarcoidosis?

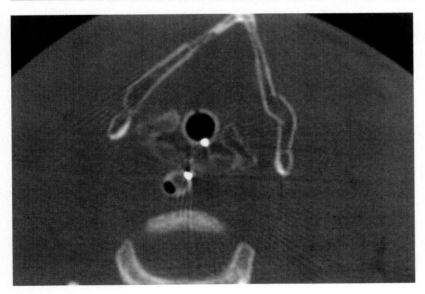

1. Which cartilage is critical for airway patency?

2. What is the most common site of traumatic laryngeal dislocations?

3. At what location do most cases of posttraumatic laryngeal stenoses occur?

4. What form of inflammatory arthritis most commonly affects the cricoarytenoid or cricothyroid joints?

Normal Facial Nerve Enhancement

1. Seventy-six percent of the time.

2. Forty-five percent of the time.

3. Hearing loss.

4. The facial nerve.

Reference

Gebarski SS, Telian SA, Niparki JK: Enhancement along the normal facial nerve in the facial canal: MR imaging and anatomic correlation, *Radiology* 183:391-394, 1992.

Cross-Reference

Neuroradiology: THE REQUISITES, pp 348-349.

Comment

Gebarski and colleagues have shown that facial nerve enhancement is the norm in most individuals because of the circumneural arteriovenous plexus in the facial nerve's tympanic and intramastoid portions. Therefore just because you see tympanic or intramastoid facial nerve enhancement in a patient with Bell's palsy, that does not mean it is abnormal, even if it is asymmetric (seen in 45% of normals). I call abnormal enhancement when the intracanalicular or intralabyrinthine portions of the nerve enhance or if there is enlargement and enhancement of the nerve in the intramastoid and tympanic portions of the nerve. At the geniculate ganglion, enhancement is almost always seen.

When should you image a patient who has features of a Bell's palsy (i.e., atypical Bell's)? Usually if the patient's symptoms have not resolved by 4 to 8 weeks after onset or if any other cranial nerves are involved, imaging with MRI is recommended.

Notes

Fracture Thyroid Cartilage

1. Cricoid cartilage.

2. At the cricoarytenoid joint.

3. The subglottic level.

4. Rheumatoid arthritis. Infections (tuberculosis most commonly) rarely affect these joints.

Reference

Hanft K, Posternack C, Astor F, Attarian D: Diagnosis and management of laryngeal trauma in sports, *South Med J* 89:631-633, 1996.

Cross-Reference

Neuroradiology: THE REQUISITES, pp 395-398.

Comment

Only 1 in 650 facial fractures affects the larynx. These days, most cases of laryngeal trauma are associated with car accidents, falls, and high velocity (biking, hockey puck) sports injuries—previously, war-related injuries dominated. Blunt injuries are 6 times more common than penetrating ones. The laryngeal flap attachment to the face masks used by many goalies in hockey games is a testament to the effects of a round missile hurtling toward one's neck. Emphysema in the neck suggests a mucosal tear of the pharynx or larynx but more commonly emanates from a pneumomediastinum. Once the mucosal surface has been denuded, the potential for infection is high, and prompt therapy is required. Mucosal grafting to cover exposed cartilage seems to be the current standard of care. Skin grafting is another option. Reconstruction of displaced bony fragments and relocation of dislocated cartilaginous junctions provide for a better outcome. The radiologist should take note of mucosal edema, extraluminal air, cricoarytenoid dislocation, and arytenoid swelling. The earlier the patient is treated, the better the ultimate outcome.

Notes

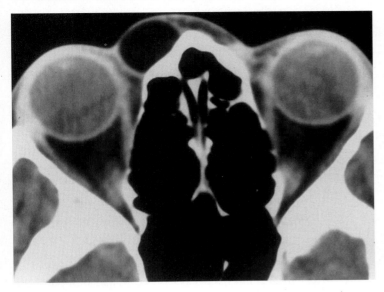
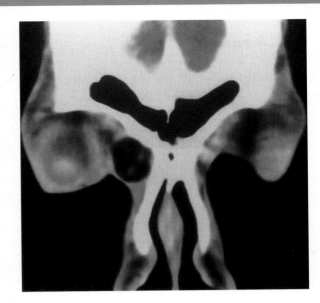

1. What are the most common sites of dermoids in the head and neck?

2. Where do midline skull dermoids occur?

3. What is the path of a dermal sinus tract to the brain?

4. How often are nasal dermoids confined to the skin and subcutaneous tissues?

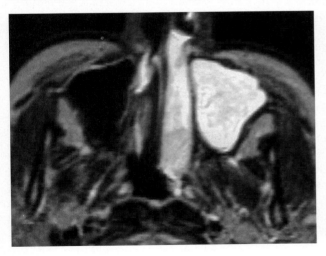
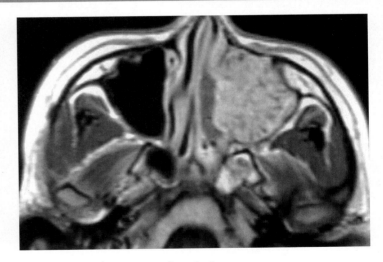

1. After squamous cell carcinoma, what malignancies are common in the sinonasal cavity?

2. Define Ohngren's line. Why is it important?

3. Where do hemangiopericytomas of the head and neck occur?

4. Where do myxomas of the head and neck occur?

Nasal Dermoid Cyst

1. The orbits, skull, tongue, anterior cervical region, and thyroid gland.

2. From most to least common—the anterior fontanelle, occiput, glabella, nasion, and vertex.

3. From the bridge of the nose through the nasal bones, across the nasal septum and cribriform plate through the crista galli, and across the leaves of the falx to the intradural compartment.

4. Over 60% of the time.

Reference

Smirniotopoulos JG, Chiechi MV: Teratomas, dermoids, and epidermoids of the head and neck, *Radiographics* 15:1437-1455, 1995.

Cross-Reference

Neuroradiology: THE REQUISITES, pp 76-77, 300, 362.

Comment

Failure of separation of surface ectoderm from underlying structures (often the neuroectoderm) is the most common explanation for the cause of epidermoids and dermoids. At the time of closure of the frontonasal groove, the nasooptic groove, or the frontal sutures a dermoid/epidermoid can occur. Whereas epidermoids are filled with keratinous debris and cholesterol, dermoids may truly have fatty material, calcification, and proteinaceous material within them. They occur most commonly around the orbits, in the skin, or in the subcutaneous tissue. Dermoids of the orbit frequent the lacrimal fossa, and they account for the majority of congenital lesions of the orbit. Fat-fluid levels, when present, are pathognomonic for a dermoid cyst. Inflammation around a dermoid may be present if it has a tract to the skin that becomes infected or if the dermoid ruptures and a chemical cellulitis from the cyst's contents ensues. The differential diagnosis of a lesion in this location (for the clinician) includes a nasal glioma, a cephalocele, a hemangioma, and a soft tissue neoplasm.

Notes

Adenoid Cystic Carcinoma of the Maxillary Sinus

1. Bone metastases, minor salivary gland tumors (adenoid cystic carcinoma, adenocarcinoma), lymphoma, sarcomas, myeloma (plasmacytoma), olfactory neuroblastomas, and melanomas.

2. It goes from the medial canthus of the eye to the angle of the mandible and divides the maxillary sinus into a posterosuperior and anteroinferior compartment. Tumors that are anteroinferior have a better prognosis owing to less orbital, intracranial, and skull base involvement.

3. Most are in the sinonasal cavity.

4. Most occur in the mandible, followed by the hard palate.

Reference

Chow JM, Leonetti JP, Mafee MF: Epithelial tumors of the paranasal sinuses and nasal cavity, *Radiol Clin North Am* 31:61-73, 1993.

Cross-Reference

Neuroradiology: THE REQUISITES, pp 384, 422.

Comment

Minor salivary gland neoplasms are particularly common around the palate, the nasal cavity, and the ethmoid sinuses, with less of a predilection for the maxillary sinus. Of the minor salivary gland tumors, adenoid cystic carcinoma and mucoepidermoid carcinoma dominate the rankings. Nonetheless, they represent less than 10% of all head and neck (and sinonasal) malignancies. With each and every adenoid cystic carcinoma of the head and neck, allow your eyes to stray to the pterygopalatine fossa. Invariably, where you should only see fat, teeny-tiny vessels, and the pterygopalatine ganglion you will find a discernible mass or obliterated fat. You must train yourself to look here because this area is frequently overlooked and is a common route of spread of facial malignancies.

I like to show this case because it represents the exception to the rule that something bright on a T2W scan is benign. Just looking at the T2W scan (on the left), you might think this is a patient with an opacified maxillary sinus from inflammatory disease. The contrast-enhanced scan (on the right) shows solid enhancement, which would be most unusual for anything inflammatory except for rip-roaring polyposis. The enhanced scan should definitely make you worry about a neoplasm, though with the bright T2W scan you probably thought it could be a pleomorphic adenoma. But, lo and behold, this is a high grade adenoid cystic carcinoma of a mixed tubular and cribriform type.

Notes

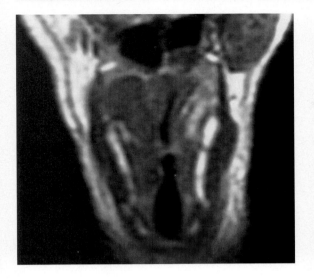 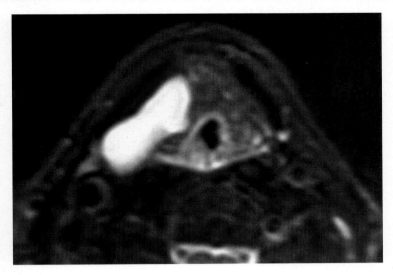

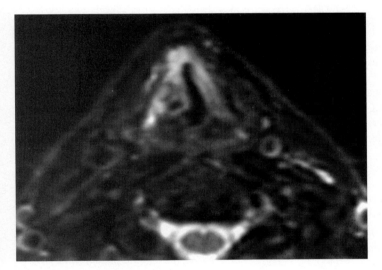

1. When cancer occurs in association with laryngoceles, where is the epicenter?

2. What is the term used for an infected laryngocele?

3. How often is cancer associated with laryngoceles?

4. What is the difference between a laryngocele, a saccular cyst, and a laryngeal mucocele?

Saccular Cyst with Laryngeal Carcinoma

1. The laryngeal ventricle.

2. Laryngopyocele.

3. Fifteen percent of the time.

4. Air is in the laryngocele, and fluid is in the saccular cyst and laryngeal mucocele. (These terms are used interchangeably.)

Reference

Harvey M, Ibrahim H, Yousem DM, Weinstein GS: Radiologic findings in a carcinoma-associated laryngocele, *Ann Otol Rhinol Laryngol* 105:405-408, 1996.

Cross-Reference

Neuroradiology: THE REQUISITES, pp 398-403.

Comment

Internal laryngoceles occur more commonly than external ones, and often the patients either are asymptomatic or have a minor voice change. There is a huge variation in the reported incidence of carcinoma in association with laryngoceles, ranging as high as 58.3% and as low as 4.9%. Laryngoceles develop in 17.8% to 28.8% (nearly 3 times the rate in the asymptomatic population) of patients with squamous cell carcinomas of the larynx. Of tumors associated with laryngoceles, supraglottic cancers (because the supraglottis includes the false cords and ventricle) are most common.

Early T1 or T2 squamous cell carcinomas of the glottis may be treated with radiation therapy or with surgery. Although the overall cure rate with radiation is slightly less than that with definitive surgery (vertical hemilaryngectomy or supracricoid laryngectomy), the voice quality and early morbidity are usually better with radiotherapy. The patients who fail radiation treatment often (80%) must go on to total laryngectomy. Overall, 50% of patients who fail radiation therapy will die of local (laryngeal) disease.

Notes

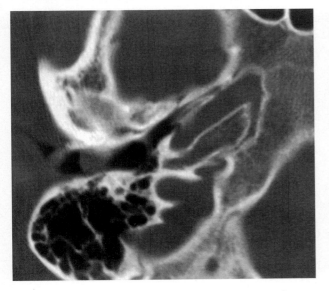
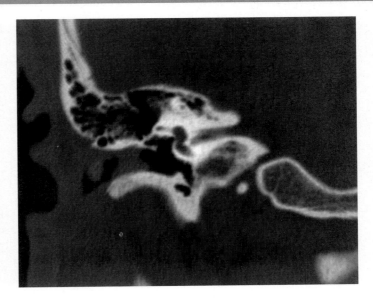

1. What are the benign soft tissue masses in the ear?

2. Name benign tumors of ceruminous gland origin.

3. Name malignant tumors of ceruminous gland origin.

4. What is the most common malignancy of the external ear?

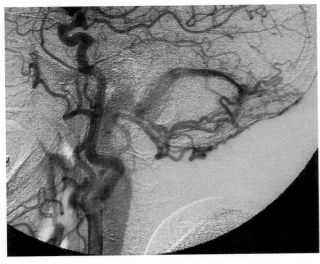
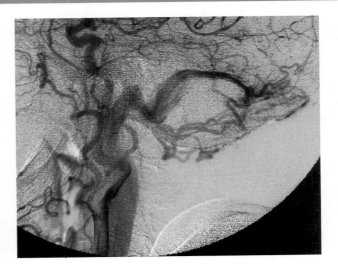

1. What is the cause of tinnitus in this patient?

2. What is the most common site of a dural arteriovenous malformation?

3. What angiographic findings suggest a higher risk of intracranial hemorrhage from dural vascular malformation?

4. What is the etiology of a dural arteriovenous malformation?

CASE 114

Polyp in Ear

1. Cholesteatomas, keratosis obturans, pleomorphic adenomas, benign polyps, epidermoids, and cerumen impactions.

2. Adenoma and pleomorphic adenoma.

3. Adenoid cystic carcinoma and adenocarcinoma are the two most common histologies.

4. Skin cancer—squamous cell or basal cell carcinoma.

Reference

Chakeres DW, Kapila A, LaMasters D: Soft-tissue abnormalities of the external auditory canal: subject review of CT findings, *Radiology* 156:105-109, 1985.

Cross-Reference

Neuroradiology: THE REQUISITES, pp 336-338.

Comment

The differential diagnosis of benign soft tissue external auditory canal tumors includes hemangiomas, papillomas, hamartomas, and the "ceruminomas" listed in answer 2. Exostoses are also common but hardly "soft tissue." Congenital epidermoid lesions or acquired cholesteatomas (particularly in individuals with external auditory canal stenosis) may present with a pearly white external auditory canal mass. It is my impression that all of these masses are a lot less common than cerumen impactions and exostoses. They are hard to differentiate radiographically except by their enhancement characteristics—only hemangiomas, adenomas, ceruminomas, and minor salivary gland tumors enhance.

Because it is such a fulminant yet treatable disease, rule out MOE any time you see an external auditory canal mass. Look for the cardinal signs of bone erosion, skull base invasion, and obliteration of parapharyngeal fat planes because the nature of the lesion in the ear may not be evident to the unwary clinician. MOE is one disease you do not want to miss—a delay in diagnosis can lead to death from diabetic ketoacidosis and sepsis.

Notes

CASE 115

Dural Arteriovenous Malformation

1. A dural arteriovenous malformation—note the early draining vein.

2. Along the walls of the sigmoid-transverse sinus.

3. Cortical venous drainage, larger size, and retrograde filling of sinuses or veins.

4. Most people believe it occurs as a result of dural thrombosis with subsequent incorporation of venous flow into an arteriovenous network along the walls of the thrombosed sinus.

Reference

Cognard C, Gobin VP, Pierot L, Bailly A-L, Houdart E, Casasco A, Chiras J, Merland J-J: Cerebral dural arteriovenous fistulas: clinical and angiographic correlation with a revised classification of venous drainage, *Radiology* 194:671-680, 1995.

Cross-Reference

Neuroradiology: THE REQUISITES, pp 496-498.

Comment

Intracranial dural AVFs may be totally asymptomatic or may cause death. Fistulas that drain with antegrade flow into a large dural sinus (and particularly the transverse or sigmoid sinus) have a benign prognosis, whereas those that drain directly into cortical veins and are associated with venous ectasia (or aneurysms) and retrograde flow have a much higher rate of intracranial hemorrhage. Any time there is reversal of flow in or drainage to veins and not sinuses, the potential for intracranial complications arises. The most common sites of dural fistulas are in the posterior fossa and the cavernous sinus. Thus tinnitus and orbital symptoms, respectively, may bring the patient to the clinician. With supratentorial dural arteriovenous malformations, symptoms of increased intracranial pressure, seizures, altered mental status, focal deficits, and hemorrhage become manifest. Dural malformations at the tentorium cerebelli, anterior cranial fossa, and torcula do worse than those elsewhere.

Half of dural AVFs occur in the posterior fossa, and dural ones make up over one third of *all* arteriovenous malformations in the posterior fossa and one tenth of *all* arteriovenous malformations in the brain. Two thirds of all arteriovenous malformations drain to either the sigmoid or transverse sinus. This case shows numerous branches of the occipital artery, stylomastoid tributaries, and other anterior feeders draining into a faintly opacified sigmoid sinus (best seen in the figure on right, in which the jugular vein is being filled as well). Venous opacification this early in the injection is pathologic.

Notes

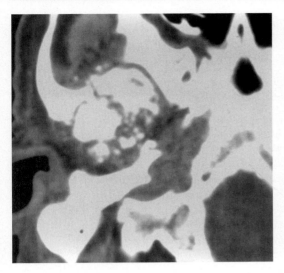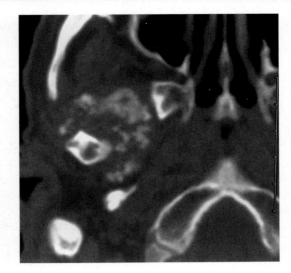

1. In the absence of a soft tissue mass associated with this lesion, what are the two best diagnoses?

2. In the presence of multiple joints exhibiting similar pathology, what should be considered?

3. What are the imaging features of pigmented villonodular synovitis on MRI?

4. What are the MRI findings of avascular necrosis of the condylar head?

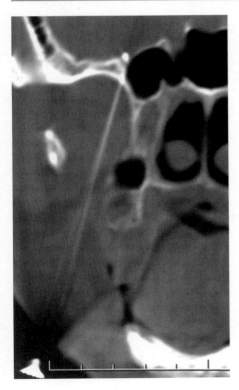

1. Through what orifice has this needle passed?

2. What is the curved wire extending out of the needle tip?

3. In what part of Meckel's cave are the mandibular nerve fibers?

4. Where is the carotid artery relative to Meckel's cave?

Synovial Chondromatosis

1. Synovial chondromatosis and chondroid tumor of the temporal bone.

2. Gout, pseudogout (crystalline calcium pyrophosphate disease), multiple chondromas, and tumoral calcinosis.

3. Hemorrhagic by-products abound. Erosive changes of bone and cartilage with cystic changes may be seen. The lesion is usually dark on T2W scans owing to hemosiderin.

4. Early on one sees dark signal intensity on T1W scans and bright signal intensity on T2W scans, presumably because of edema. With chronicity the signal decreases on T1W and T2W scans, and sclerosis is seen on CT and plain films.

Reference
Sledz K, Ortiz O, Wax M, Bouquot J: Tumoral calcinosis of the temporomandibular joint: CT and MR findings, *AJNR Am J Neuroradiol* 16:782-785, 1995.

Cross-Reference
Neuroradiology: THE REQUISITES, pp 424-427.

Comment
Synovial chondromatosis is characterized by synovial metaplasia with intraarticular loose body formation. These loose bodies appear as multiple densities in and around the joint. The entity is more commonly monoarticular and is seen in young adults (mean age 46, women > men). Pain is a component of the disease. The larger joints are more commonly affected than the small ones. The differential diagnosis includes tumoral calcinosis, which produces large periarticular calcified masses, though the temporomandibular joint is a lot less frequently involved than hips, elbows, and shoulders. Tumoral calcinosis is seen in young African Americans. Other entities to be considered include calcium pyrophosphate deposition disease, chronic renal failure with dystrophic calcification, dialysis arthropathy, and chondroosseous neoplasms.

Notes

Trigeminal Nerve Neurolysis

1. The foramen ovale.

2. A thermocoagulation electrode used for neurolysis.

3. The inferolateral portion of the cavity. (Sensory V-3 fibers are lateral to motor V-3 ones.)

4. Medial and anterior.

Reference
Majoie CB, Verbeeten B Jr, Dol JA, Peeters FL: Trigeminal neuropathy: evaluation with MR imaging, *Radiographics* 15:795-811, 1995.

Cross-Reference
Neuroradiology: THE REQUISITES, p 51.

Comment
It only took me an hour and a half of manipulating to get the needle into Meckel's cave, despite how easy this looks on the CT scan. The patient had trigeminal neuralgia and was not a surgical candidate, and I wanted to guide the needle under CT rather than fluoroscopy, though the latter may have been easier in retrospect. Surgeons place needles through the foramen ovale under fluoroscopic guidance frequently—in fact, a neurosurgical resident snickered at me when he walked in during this procedure.

Multiple sclerosis is one of the most common causes of trigeminal neuropathy and was the cause of pain in this patient. Otherwise, one should consider infarcts and gliomas in the brain stem. Tic douloureux (trigeminal neuralgia) is most frequently caused by vascular compression of the fifth cranial nerve (especially V-2 and V-3) and is usually due to compression from the superior cerebellar artery, inferior cerebellar artery, vertebral artery, or basilar artery. Venous compression may also occur, and still other causes appear to be from microvascular compression by tiny arterial or venous branches. In any case, decompression appears to work, whether it be arterial, venous, or capillary. Beware that 30% of normal asymptomatic patients have what appears to be vascular compression of the root entry zone of the trigeminal nerve.

Notes

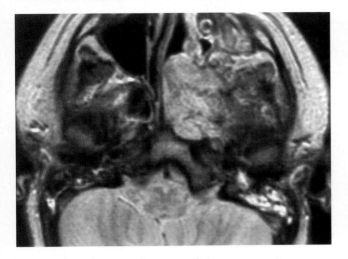 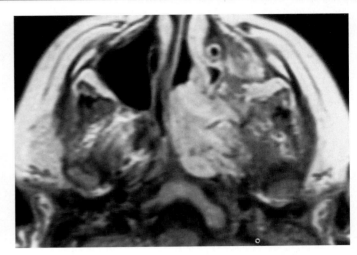

1. What is the site of origin of these tumors?

2. What are the staging issues?

3. What are classic symptoms?

4. What is the treatment?

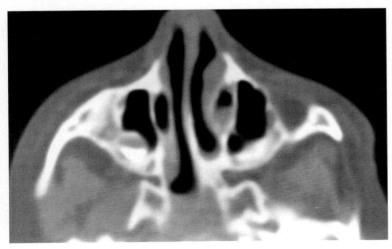

1. What is the breakdown between bony and fibrous choanal atresia?

2. How do unilateral choanal atresia and bilateral choanal atresia differ in presentation?

3. What are the associated anomalies for which one should look?

4. Which is more common, unilateral or bilateral choanal atresia?

CASE 118

Juvenile Angiofibroma

1. It is controversial. The nasopharynx, the pterygopalatine fossa, the sphenopalatine foramen, the masticator space, the posterior end of the middle turbinate—all of these have been proposed. I say the sphenopalatine foramen. Trust me!

2. Spread intracranially or into the orbit (grade 3), into the pterygopalatine fossa or masticator space (grade 2), or confined to the nasopharynx (grade 1).

3. Recurrent epistaxis and nasal fullness in a teenaged boy.

4. Preoperative embolization and definitive surgery.

Reference

Berger SB, Chaloupka JC, Putman CM, Citardi MJ, Lamb T, Sasaki CL: Hypervascular tumor of the buccal space in an adult as a late recurrence of juvenile angiofibroma, *AJNR Am J Neuroradiol* 17:1384-1387, 1996.

Cross-Reference

Neuroradiology: THE REQUISITES, p 380.

Comment

This is a disease of adolescent boys, with classic imaging features of anterior bowing of the posterior wall of the maxillary antrum (99%), widening of the pterygopalatine fossa (90%), and a densely enhancing mass fed predominantly by ascending pharyngeal branches. Flow voids are often identified on MRI. Intracranial disease occurs in up to 20% of cases via the foramina of the pterygopalatine fossa (vidian canal, foramen rotundum). Occasionally the tumor blasts through the junction of the pterygoid bone and the body of the sphenoid bone to extend intracranially into the middle cranial fossa.

Outside the nasopharynx, the most common sites of angiofibromas are the maxillary and ethmoid sinuses. Juvenile angiofibromas in females are rare but not impossible to find, particularly if extrapharyngeal. A hormonal influence appears to be at play here.

Although surgical treatment (after endovascular embolization) is preferred, radiation is also effective at relatively low doses (<4000 rad). Remember that this is a benign though aggressive tumor, so arrest of growth rather than disfiguring, high-morbidity curative surgery may be the way to go.

Notes

CASE 119

Choanal Atresia (Bony on Left)

1. Bony 90%, membranous 10%. (I think these bony numbers are high!) Many people include the classification of a "mixed" bony and membranous form, which may account for the majority of the types previously classified as "bony."

2. Bilateral choanal atresia presents in neonates at birth because infants are obligate nose breathers. Unilateral choanal atresia may not be evident until adulthood and may masquerade as chronic sinusitis.

3. CHARGE syndrome (coloboma, heart defects, choanal atresia, mental retardation, genital hypoplasia, and ear anomalies), Treacher Collins syndrome (jaw and ear anomalies), and skull base anomalies.

4. Unilateral.

Reference

Rothman G, Wood RA, Naclerio RM: Unilateral choanal atresia masquerading as chronic sinusitis, *Pediatrics* 946:941-944, 1994.

Cross-Reference

Neuroradiology: THE REQUISITES, pp 362-363.

Comment

Unilateral choanal atresia is a diagnosis that one should always consider while evaluating coronal or axial sinus CT scans for unilateral sinusitis. Mucous discharge from that nasal aperture may be limited. Choanal atresia is the most common congenital nasal anomaly, usually reported in 1 out of 5000 to 10,000 births and more common in females. There is a higher rate in white children but no clear gender or right-left predilections. California has the highest rate of occurrence in the United States. Chromosomal anomalies are found in 6% of infants with choanal atresia, and 5% of patients with choanal atresia have a documented genetic syndrome.

Axial CT scans should be performed after suctioning and application of decongestants, lest mucosal thickening be mistaken for fibrous obliteration of the nasal cavity. CT should describe the site, thickness, side, and type of obstruction. The nasal cavity is usually narrowed, with deformity of the vomer and an enlarged nasopharyngeal airway.

Choanal atresia has most recently been treated endoscopically to punch a hole through to the airway. Three-dimensional intraoperative guidance and imaging may be helpful to the surgeon when using this technique.

Notes

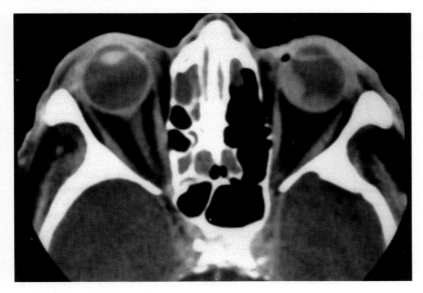

1. What are the common causes of choroidal detachment?

2. What is ocular hypotony?

3. What is the ora serrata, and how does it help distinguish choroidal versus retinal detachments?

4. How are the shapes of choroidal effusions and hematomas different?

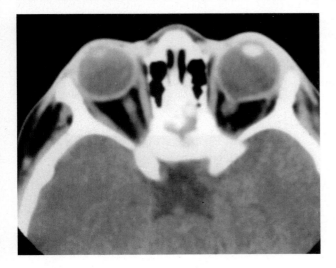

1. What is the cause of a coloboma?

2. What are the intracranial associations?

3. What are the clinical findings?

4. What are the predisposing factors?

Choroidal Detachment, Lens Implant

1. Iatrogenic after surgery, trauma, infection, and neoplasms.

2. A state in which the intraocular pressure drops, thereby predisposing to a choroidal effusion as the globe sinks in, pulling fluid out of choroidal capillaries.

3. It is the anterior termination of the retina proximal to the ciliary body. Whereas choroidal detachments (because the choroid goes up to the ciliary body) cross the ora serrata, retinal detachments do not cross it and stop proximal to the iris and ciliary muscles.

4. Effusions are ring or crescent-shaped, whereas hematomas are lenticular (like subdural versus epidural intracranial hematomas).

Reference

Mafee MF, Linder B, Peyman GA, Langer BG, Choi KH, Capek V: Choroidal hematoma and effusion: evaluation with MR imaging, *Radiology* 168:781-786, 1988.

Cross-Reference

Neuroradiology: THE REQUISITES, pp 287-288.

Comment

Choroidal detachments may be serous or hemorrhagic. Most choroidal hematomas (hemorrhagic choroidal detachments) are due to significant trauma to the globe with a clot in its wall. The blood products evolve like epidural hematomas of the brain—slowly. Serous choroidal detachments (choroidal effusions) are less dramatic and may be seen as tiny peripheral collections along the edges of the globe. Exudation of fluid from uveitis can cause choroidal effusions. Effusions are usually bright on all MRI pulse sequences owing to protein effects.

The differential diagnosis in this case includes choroidal neoplasms such as melanomas (which may cause choroidal detachments), metastases, and hemangiomas. I believe this case occurred in the perioperative setting of the lens implantation surgery.

Notes

Left Optic Nerve Coloboma

1. Incomplete closure of the choroidal fissure of the eye.

2. Agenesis of the corpus callosum and encephaloceles.

3. Leukokoria and excavation of the optic disk—morning glory syndrome.

4. It is inherited as an autosomal dominant disorder and is bilateral in 60% of patients.

Reference

Murphy BL, Griffin JF: Optic nerve coloboma (morning glory syndrome): CT findings, *Radiology* 191:59-61, 1994.

Cross-Reference

Neuroradiology: THE REQUISITES, p 289.

Comment

This disorder may be accompanied by microphthalmia, optic nerve atrophy, blindness, and strabismus. The invagination into the optic nerve may be variable in degree. Scleral thinning on CT is evident, and the globe assumes a nonspheric shape. The invagination into the optic nerve head region looks like a small cyst with vitreous humor density.

The differential diagnosis of a misshapen globe with posterior protrusion includes a staphyloma, axial myopia, congenital glaucoma, and a coloboma. Staphylomas show thinning of the scleral-choroidal membranes and are often eccentric to the optic nerve insertion site. They may coexist with severe axial myopia. Severe axial myopia is seen as an oblong oval-shaped globe with smooth symmetric scleral membranes, and the patients have severe near-sightedness. Buphthalmos (cow's eye) and congenital glaucoma are terms used synonymously and are due to an intraocular pressure–related effect that is the result of anterior chamber angle obstruction in the eye.

Notes

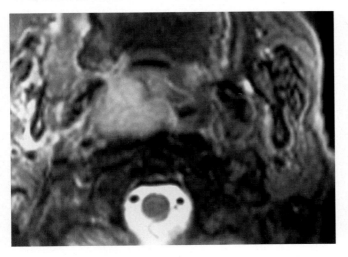 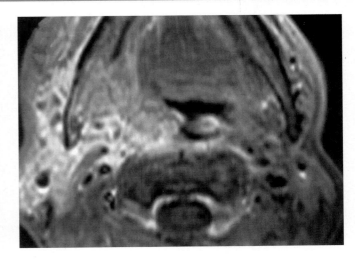

1. What is the most common tumor to invade the retropharyngeal space?

2. What are the most common primary sites of squamous cell carcinoma that invade the retropharyngeal compartment?

3. What is the significance of fixation of tumor to the prevertebral muscles (longus colli, longus capitis)?

4. What is the best criterion for determining absence of invasion of the prevertebral muscles or fascia?

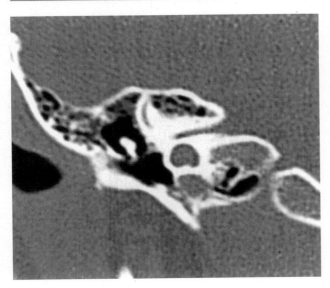 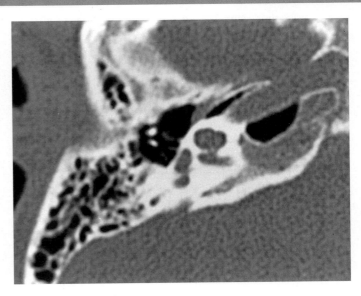

1. What percentage of all inner ear malformations are due to Mondini deformity?

2. What is the last semicircular canal (and therefore the one with the highest rate of congenital maldevelopment) to form?

3. What is the Mondini malformation?

4. How wide is the normal endolymphatic sac?

Retropharyngeal Space Invasion by Pharyngeal Carcinoma

1. Squamous cell carcinoma.

2. Nasopharynx and oropharynx.

3. It makes the tumor unresectable.

4. Preservation of the retropharyngeal fat plane.

Reference

Loevner LA, Ott II, Yousem DM, Montone KT, Thaler ER, Chalian AA, Weinstein GS, Weber RS: Neoplastic fixation to the prevertebral compartment by squamous cell carcinoma of the head and neck: correlation of MR imaging with panendoscopy and intraoperative assessment, *AJR Am J Roentgenol* 170:1998.

Cross-Reference

Neuroradiology: THE REQUISITES, pp 433-435.

Comment

Unfortunately, imaging is not very accurate in predicting prevertebral muscle or fascial invasion. On MRI neither effacement of the fat, indentation of the prevertebral muscles, serrated border to the muscle, abnormal T2W signal in the muscle, nor enhancement of the muscle accurately predicts singularly or in combination whether the prevertebral musculature is invaded. This is an important point because if MRI could positively predict invasion it would obviate the need for an "open and close" surgical procedure in which the oncologic surgeon finds, belatedly, that the patient is inoperable because of prevertebral invasion. The surgeon tries to manipulate the tumor off the muscles manually or create a plane with his or her finger to see if the tumor is removable. The surgeon cannot simply resect the prevertebral muscles. Unfortunately, those muscles are necessary to flex and rotate the head, so they are indispensable. The patient is therefore stuck with inoperable cancer or an operation after which his or her head falls off. Actually, the usual treatment in these cases is radiation therapy, but prognosis is poor.

To reiterate, the demarcation between the nasopharynx and the oropharynx along the posterior pharyngeal wall is the plane parallel to the hard palate–soft palate junction. Because this case is below the hard palate and the lesion appears to also invade the soft palate proper and tonsil, I would say this lesion arose in the oropharynx. This is not to say that a nasopharynx cancer cannot grow down to the oropharynx (fairly common) or that an oropharyngeal primary tumor cannot grow superiorly to the nasopharynx (a little less common).

Notes

Mondini Malformation*

1. Fifty-five percent.

2. The lateral semicircular canal.

3. An incomplete number of turns of the cochlea.

4. Less than or equal to 1.5 mm.

Reference

Urman SM, Talbot JM: Otic capsule dysplasia: clinical and CT findings, *Radiographics* 10:823-838, 1990.

Cross-Reference

Neuroradiology: THE REQUISITES, p 349.

Comment

There are varying degrees of cochlear malformations—from complete aplasia (bone fills in the spot) to single cavity cochlea (no internal architecture to the turns of the cochlea) to the Mondini malformation (incomplete development of the middle and apical turns of the cochlea). On the vestibular side, the fewer and less mature the semicircular canals are, the larger the vestibule is. The lateral semicircular canal is affected most commonly because it develops last. Michel's aplasia affects both cochlear and vestibular systems and is thought to result from an arrest of development in the fourth week of fetal development. You see a common cavity between the vestibular and cochlear systems.

Normal development of the internal ear structures starts with an otic placode derived from neuroectoderm. The placode invaginates to form an otic pit, which seals off as an otic vesicle. The structure elongates medially with protrusions for the endolymphatic sac and semicircular canals. Anteriorly there is an evagination for the cochlear duct, which by the eighth week of gestation spirals around to form the normal nautilus configuration of the cochlea. The central cavity then divides into the utricle and saccule of the vestibular system.

Notes

---

* Figures for Case 123 courtesy Azita Khorsandi, MD.

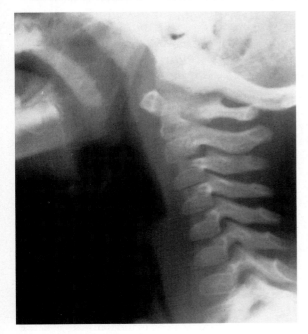

1. What are the common causes of subglottic stenosis in neonates?

2. What is the usual course of the disease?

3. At what minimal diameter should one intervene to correct neonatal airway stenosis?

4. What study best evaluates the patient for subglottic stenosis?

CASE 125

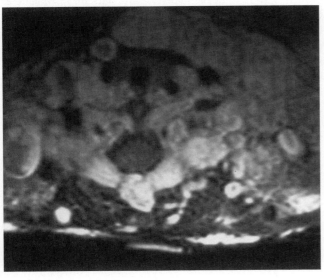 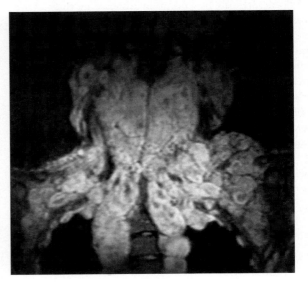

1. Which type of NF is more likely to show plexiform neurofibromas?

2. Are plexiform neurofibromas found peripherally or centrally?

3. Where are the most common sites of neurofibromas in the head and neck region?

4. What bone dysplasia may be seen with NF type 1 and plexiform neurofibromas of the orbit?

Subglottic Stenosis*

1. Congenital weakness, hemangiomas, iatrogenesis (after intubation), Down syndrome, and tracheoesophageal fistula.

2. When idiopathic, it resolves on its own.

3. A diameter of 3.5 mm.

4. Videofluoroscopy.

Reference

Rimell FL, Stool SE: Diagnosis and management of pediatric tracheal stenosis, *Otolaryngol Clin North Am* 28:809-827, 1995.

Cross-Reference

Neuroradiology: THE REQUISITES, p 397.

Comment

In children one should consider vascular slings (pulmonary artery sling, double aortic arch, and so on), extrinsic vascular compressions (innominate artery causing anterior tracheal compression), papillomatosis, minor salivary gland tumors, rhabdomyomas, pulmonary hypertension, and mediastinal tumors in the differential diagnosis of lower airway stenosis. In the upper airway, cricoid stenosis, laryngomalacia, and primary tracheal stenosis may be at work. More commonly the stenosis is acquired as a result of endotracheal tube intubations with development of perichondritis. Webs and synechiae may follow. Gastroesophageal reflux exacerbates the stenosis by inducing continued inflammation and irritation.

Subglottic stenosis can occur in association with Down syndrome and Wegener's granulomatosis. One theory regarding the cause of idiopathic subglottic stenosis proposes that there is an autoimmune attack on the cricoid cartilage leading to or resulting from subglottic inflammation, degradation of the extracellular matrix, and exposure of cricoid collagen to immunologic attack. Still others believe fibrogenic peptides mediate the fibrotic reaction in the subglottis. The main role of the imager is to exclude a mass, ring, or sling as the cause of the stenosis.

Notes

Plexiform Neurofibroma

1. Type 1.

2. Peripherally.

3. The eyelids, orbit, cheek, and nose.

4. Absence or hypoplasia of the greater sphenoid wing.

Reference

Sobol SE, Tewfik TL, Ortenberg J: Otolaryngologic manifestations of neurofibromatosis in children, *J Otolaryngol* 26:13-20, 1997.

Cross-Reference

Neuroradiology: THE REQUISITES, p 267.

Comment

Head and neck manifestations (excluding intracranial lesions) occur in 14% to 22% of individuals with NF. The chief complaints are usually due to pigmentary changes, neurofibromas, and bony dysplasias, with cosmetic deformities leading the pack. However, an enlarging neck or orbital mass affecting vision or hearing can also be a primary presentation of children with NF type 1. The plexiform neurofibroma is one of the seven diagnostic criteria for NF type 1 (six or more café au lait spots, two or more neurofibromas, axillary or inguinal freckling, optic pathway glioma, two or more Lisch nodules, an osseous lesion, and a first degree relative with the disease). In the head and neck, cranial nerves III, V, VII, and IX are the most common to be affected, but cervical spinal nerve plexiform neurofibromas are just as common. The entire nerve is infiltrated by the neurofibroma, and it may be hypervascular and may simulate a hemangioma. This is one of the lesions that does not respect the fascial planes of the spaces of the head and neck. Plexiform neurofibromas show a disordered array of Schwann cells with fibroblasts, collagen, and a loose matrix infiltrating multiple fascicles and axons of the nerve histopathologically. The risk of malignant degeneration is substantial (13% to 30%). Nine percent of all individuals with neurofibromas have von Recklinghausen's disease, and most neurofibromas are solitary. Neurofibromas are a lot less common than schwannomas.

Notes

---

* Figure for Case 124 courtesy Hervey D. Segall, MD, and Marvin D. Nelson, Jr., MD.

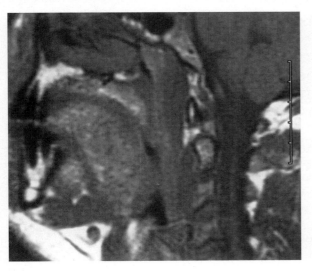 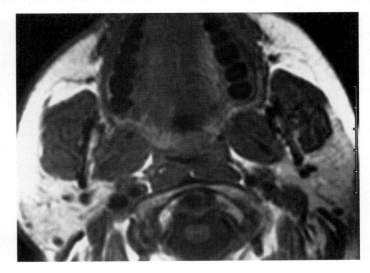

1. Where is the most common site of obstruction in patients with sleep apnea syndrome?

2. How narrow is a narrow pharyngeal cross-section?

3. What is the usual treatment for obstructive sleep apnea syndrome?

4. Who is Pickwick of pickwickian syndrome?

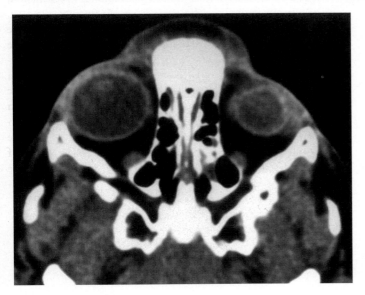

1. What are the two most common causes of leukokoria in childhood?

2. Is the globe big or small with persistent hyperplastic primary vitreous (PHPV)?

3. What is the vessel and canal that fails to regress with PHPV?

4. Does PHPV calcify?

Sleep Apnea

1. At the uvula–soft palate level.

2. Less than 50 mm² cross-sectional area for severe sleep apnea, and 50 to 100 mm² for moderate sleep apnea.

3. Uvulotonsillopalatopharyngoplasty (or variations of the procedure).

4. Samuel Pickwick is a character in the novel *The Posthumous Papers of the Pickwick Club* by Charles Dickens. Pickwick is described as fat, red-faced (probably from polycythemia), and somnolent (from interrupted sleep).

Reference

Avrahami E, Englender M: Relation between CT axial cross-sectional area of the oropharynx and obstructive sleep apnea syndrome in adults, *AJNR Am J Neuroradiol* 16:135-140, 1996.

Cross-Reference

Neuroradiology: THE REQUISITES, pp 384-388.

Comment

Not exactly one of the most exciting topics—snoring, obese, hypoxic individuals—but one that has garnered a lot of press in the past. Basically, these patients often have an abundance of floppy lymphoid tissue or mobile tongues, mandibles, maxillas, palates, and pharyngeal mucosa that intermittently obstruct the airway. Cross-sectional area measurements of the pharynx show pretty good correlations with number and duration of apneic episodes and oxygen desaturation. Airway length and height also seem to predict who will respond well to uvulopalatopharyngoplasty. Some patients also respond to intraoral mandibular repositioning devices, splints, or tongue reduction surgery.

Notes

Persistent Hyperplastic Primary Vitreous

1. Retinoblastoma and persistent hyperplastic primary vitreous.

2. Small.

3. The hyaloid artery in Cloquet's canal.

4. Usually not, but the globe is hyperdense.

Reference

Magill HL, Hanna SL, Brooks MT, Jenkins JJ III, Burton EW, Bouldler TF, Seidel FG: Case of the day: pediatric—persistent hyperplastic primary vitreous (PHPV), *Radiographics* 10:515-518, 1990.

Cross-Reference

Neuroradiology: THE REQUISITES, p 286.

Comment

The hyaloid artery, which early in gestation provides the vascular supply to the vitreous and lens, normally regresses by the seventh month of gestation. It forms Cloquet's canal, which is a nearly invisible lymphatic link from the lens to the optic nerve head. The lens is nearly always abnormal with PHPV, one of the differential diagnostic points in this entity. PHPV can lead to retinal detachment, hemorrhage into the vitreous, glaucoma, and cataract formation in an infant. That eye is blind. Enucleation often is required. The absence of calcification and the presence of microphthalmia in PHPV are the two clues in distinguishing retinoblastoma from PHPV because both entities present with leukokoria in an infant.

Microphthalmia may be seen in cases of phthisis bulbi, colobomas, and hypoplasia of the optic nerve, and it may also be seen as the residuum of intrauterine infections such as those caused by *Toxocara*. Lowe syndrome (Charles Upton Lowe, American pediatrician, 1921-?), also known as oculocerebrorenal syndrome (rickets, glaucoma, cataracts, mental retardation, and renal tubular abnormalities as an X-linked recessive trait), and oculomandibulofacial syndrome (Hallermann-Streiff-François syndrome with brachycephaly, parrot nose, mandibular hypoplasia, congenital cataracts, and dwarfism) are also associated with microphthalmia.

Notes

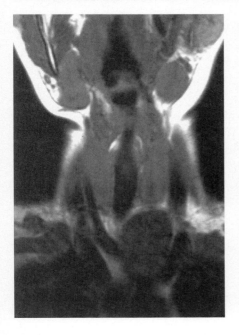
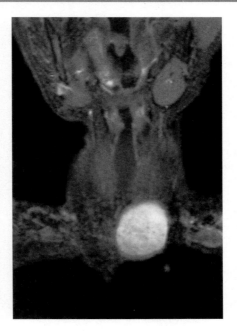

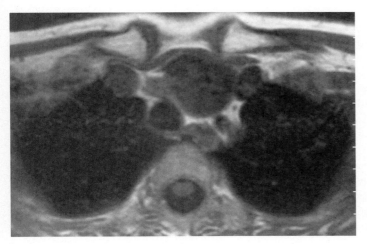

1. Are thymic cysts more common than thyroglossal duct cysts?

2. Where do thymic cysts occur?

3. With what neoplasm do thymic cysts often coexist?

4. What neurodegenerative disorder is associated with thymomas?

Thymic Cyst

1. No.

2. In the lower neck and the mediastinum.

3. Hodgkin's lymphoma.

4. Myasthenia gravis.

Reference

Nguyen Q, deTar M, Wells W, Crockett D: Cervical thymic cyst: case reports and review of the literature, *Laryngoscope* 106:247-252, 1996.

Cross-Reference

Neuroradiology: THE REQUISITES, pp 438, 444.

Comment

Thymic cysts are pretty rare. They are thought to arise congenitally from the thymopharyngeal ducts or as a result of inflammatory degeneration of the thymus. The cysts are often multiloculated, thin-walled, and paratracheal or intramediastinal. I think the coronal T1W scan best shows that this is not a thyroid lesion, but you should probably include an exophytic thyroid cyst in the differential diagnosis.

The thymus is an underrated organ in adulthood—we tend to ignore this clump of fatty tissue that, in childhood, has a major immunologic role. It develops from the third pharyngeal pouch and may extend inferiorly from its primordial connection to the inferior parathyroid glands (which also are from the third pharyngeal pouch—superior parathyroid glands, paradoxically, arise from the fourth pharyngeal pouch) and the superoanterior mediastinum.

Remember the association of thymomas and myasthenia gravis, and thymomas and red cell aplasia. The thymus may appear as a large mediastinal mass after the use of steroids or after the relief of severe body stress ("thymic rebound"). It is also enlarged in patients with hyperthyroidism, Addison's disease, lymphoma, leukemia, and Langerhans cell histiocytosis. It is absent in DiGeorge syndrome.

Notes

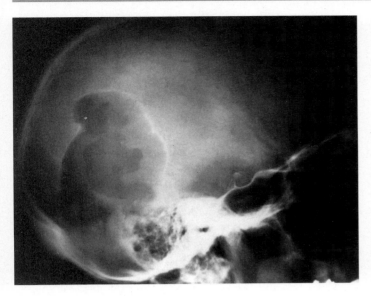 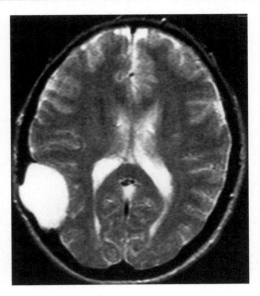

1. Why do some people consider epidermoid lesions congenital and not neoplastic?

2. How can trauma (or surgery) "cause" epidermoids?

3. Do epidermoids enhance?

4. What one sequence best differentiates between an arachnoid cyst and an epidermoid tumor?

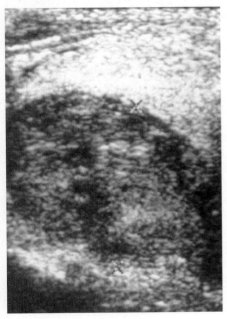

1. Which is most worrisome for thyroid malignancy—eggshell, clumped, or microcalcifications?

2. What are the ramifications of a cyst with a calcified mural nodule on ultrasound?

3. What benign inflammatory lesion of the thyroid gland most simulates a thyroid cancer?

4. What is the incidence of nodal metastases at the time of diagnosis of papillary carcinoma of the thyroid gland?

CASE 129

Calvarial Epidermoid Tumor

1. Because they arise from ectodermal inclusions during closure of the neural tube.

2. Rests of epidermal cells can be left behind in a tract, which may produce epidermal inclusion cysts.

3. Not usually.

4. FLAIR or diffusion-weighted scans (dark in cases of arachnoid cyst, bright in cases of epidermoid tumor).

Reference
Gormley WB, Tomecek FJ, Qureshi N, Malik GM: Craniocerebral epidermoid and dermoid tumours: a review of 32 cases, *Acta Neurochir* 128:115-121, 1994.

Cross-Reference
Neuroradiology: THE REQUISITES, p 77.

Comment
The calvarial epidermoid tumor (pearly tumor) is due to a rest of epithelium cells caught in the diploic space of the skull during the third to fifth weeks of gestation. The extradural epidermoids usually present as a result of local mass effect or headache, and the frontal and temporal bones are most commonly affected. The masses are hypodense on CT, with no enhancement and no vascularity on angiography. Resection of extradural epidermoids is highly successful, with a very low rate of recurrence. Dermoids usually occur in the midline, and epidermoids usually occur off midline. Posttraumatic epidermoid cysts may occur after lumbar puncture, surgery, trauma, or catheter placement. The differential diagnosis in this case may be a "leptomeningeal cyst," or so-called growing fracture, which results from posttraumatic herniation of dural membranes into a fracture site. The CSF pulsations then expand the fracture margins to create a lytic bony defect. Eosinophilic granulomas and tuberculosis of bone can simulate calvarial epidermoids on skull films.

Notes

CASE 130

Papillary Carcinoma of the Thyroid Gland (Follicular Variant)

1. Microcalcifications.

2. The possibility of papillary cystadenocarcinoma should be raised.

3. Riedel's thyroiditis.

4. Fifty percent. (Twenty-two percent of patients may have an occult primary tumor.)

Reference
Livolsi VA: Papillary neoplasms of the thyroid: pathologic and prognostic features, *Am J Clin Pathol* 97:426-434, 1992.
Yousem DM: Parathyroid and thyroid imaging, *Neuroimaging Clin N Am* 6:435-460, 1996.

Cross-Reference
Neuroradiology: THE REQUISITES, pp 438-441.

Comment
That this lesion arises from the thyroid gland is a little tricky; however, this is a thyroid ultrasound. Papillary thyroid cancer is a disease of young women—the older the age at discovery, the worse the long-term prognosis and the more likely the patient has an anaplastic variant. Also, the higher the postoperative thyroglobulin level, the worse the long-term prognosis. Papillary cancers constitute 80% of all thyroid malignancies but have a good prognosis owing to their low rate of hematogenous metastases (5% to 7%). Only 2% to 39% of resected papillary carcinomas extend beyond the thyroid capsule in surgical specimens. The follicular variant has a prognosis similar to that of traditional papillary carcinomas, and the distinction is merely made pathologically based on histologic morphology.

The factors that suggest a benign lesion on ultrasound—that is, hypoechoic borders, high echogenicity, well-defined margins, hypovascularity on pulsed Doppler evaluation, and dense calcification—are occasionally also seen with malignancies, so invariably the mass is needled.

Nodularity to the thyroid glands is found in 4% of individuals on palpation, 25% on ultrasonography, and 50% on autopsy examination. Incidence rates for occult thyroid carcinoma range between 6.5% and 35.6%. The Japanese have a particularly high rate of thyroid cancer, but North Americans have a lower rate. Anyone who has had low-dose radiation exposure (in yesteryear thymic, adenoid, and cutaneous irradiation for acne or fungal infections) is at particular risk.

Notes

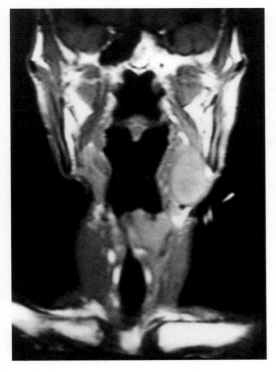
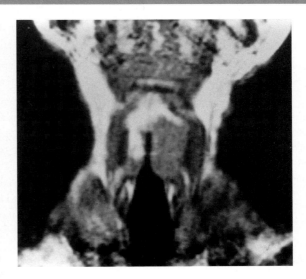

1. Where is the primary tumor located?

2. This lesion was thought to be a T1 supraglottic tumor. Why?

3. Describe T staging of supraglottic cancers.

4. What are the subsites of the supraglottis?

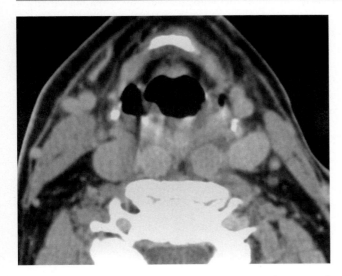

1. What are normally present in the retropharyngeal space?

2. What fasciae make up the margins of the retropharyngeal space?

3. When can carotid arteries extend medially behind the pharyngeal wall?

4. What are "kissing carotids"?

Laryngeal Carcinoma

1. In the supraglottis, with paraglottic spread.

2. Paraglottic spread is invisible to endoscopy sometimes. One subsite of the supraglottis was thought to be involved.

3. T1—tumor limited to one subsite of supraglottis, with normal vocal cord mobility; T2—tumor invades more than one subsite of supraglottis or glottis, with normal vocal cord mobility; T3—tumor limited to larynx, with vocal cord fixation, and/or tumor invades postcricoid area, medial wall of pyriform sinus, or preepiglottic tissues; and T4—tumor invades through thyroid cartilage and/or extends to other tissues beyond the larynx.

4. They include the false cords, arytenoids, suprahyoid epiglottis, infrahyoid epiglottis, and aryepiglottic folds.

Reference

Castelijns JA, van den Brekel MWM, Niekoop MM, Snow GB: Imaging of the larynx, *Neuroimaging Clin N Am* 6:401-415, 1996.

Cross-Reference

Neuroradiology: THE REQUISITES, pp 395-403.

Comment

It behooves every radiologist to learn the TNM classification of head and neck cancers or at least to hang it on the wall by the alternator for easy reference. How else can you be sure to include all of the information in the report that is helpful to the clinician to stage the disease, plan the appropriate therapy, and give an accurate estimation of the prognosis to the patient? For supraglottic cancers, be sure to assess the preepiglottic fat (suggesting T3) cancer and extension outside the larynx, which converts the tumor to a T4 category. Tumor extent to the interarytenoid region may preclude voice conservation surgery even if the cancer remains supraglottic. Tumors with bulky invasion of the preepiglottic space or ones with volumes greater than or equal to 3.5 ml are often incurable with radiation therapy alone. Paraglottic spread in the submucosal space is invisible to the clinician and may also lead to more aggressive therapy and worse morbidity for the patient.

Supraglottic cancers account for one quarter to one third of all laryngeal cancers. They are rarely discovered when they are T1 or T2 in their staging and hence have a worse prognosis than glottic cancers, which present earlier because of voice changes. Subglottic carcinomas are very uncommon. Because subglottic cancers often affect the cricoid cartilage they often necessitate total laryngectomy.

Notes

Retropharyngeal Carotid Arteries

1. Fat and lymph nodes.

2. The buccopharyngeal fascia anteriorly, the alar fascia posteriorly and laterally, and the cloison sagittale laterally.

3. When the cloison sagittale or alar fascia is incompetent. This allows medial orientation of the carotids.

4. Medial orientation of both carotids so that they "touch" in a retropharyngeal location.

Reference

Fix TJ, Daffner, RH, Deeb ZL: Carotid transposition: another cause of wide retropharyngeal soft tissues, *AJR Am J Roentgenol* 167:1305-1307, 1996.

Cross-Reference

Neuroradiology: THE REQUISITES, pp 433-435.

Comment

In the acute traumatic setting, a plain film is usually performed to assess the cervical spine. "Yikes—the retropharyngeal/precervical tissue is widened. There must be a retropharyngeal hematoma and/or a ligamentous/osseous injury to the cervical spine." The differential diagnosis of prevertebral soft tissue widening includes medial deviation of the carotid arteries, abscess, crying child's normal redundant mucosa, tumors, and swallowing artifact. A retropharyngeal carotid artery is a "gimme" on a CT scan performed for cervical spine trauma. Do not let the surgeon "drain" this "hematoma" before the CT!

Another normal variation seen in this case is asymmetry in the size of the piriform sinuses. I tend to be an under-caller. Unless I see deviation of normal structures or extramucosal growth (or unless the requisition says there is a mass there), I downplay such asymmetries and ascribe them to pooled secretions. One can always perform a "puffed out cheeks" exam of the patient with a nasopharyngolaryngoscope in the office (the mirror exam seems to be a thing of the past) or at the time of the CT to see into the piriform sinus. This is way too hard to do in the MRI magnet—puffing for the 5- to 6-minute exam may desaturate the patient!

Notes

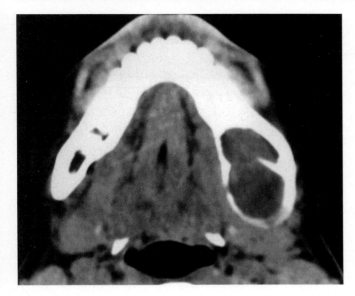

1. Are ameloblastomas more common in the mandible or in the maxilla? By how much?

2. Are ameloblastomas usually unilocular or multilocular? By how much?

3. What percent of ameloblastomas show malignant behavior?

4. Are ameloblastomas the most common cystic lesion of the mandible? What percentage do they represent?

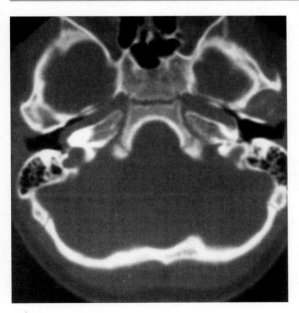

1. From what vessel does the aberrant carotid artery derive?

2. With what lesion is the aberrant carotid frequently mistaken?

3. How do patients with aberrant carotids present?

4. Is the tinnitus objective or subjective?

CASE 133

Ameloblastoma

1. Mandible by a 4:1 ratio.

2. Multilocular by a 4:1 ratio.

3. One percent.

4. No, they represent 1% of all mandibular cystic lesions.

Reference

Minami M, Kaneda T, Yamamoto H, Ozawa K, Itai Y, Ozawa M, Yoshikawa K, Sasaki Y: Ameloblastoma in the maxillo-mandibular region: MR imaging, *Radiology* 184:389-394, 1992.

Cross-Reference

Neuroradiology: THE REQUISITES, pp 391, 427.

Comment

The classic appearance of an expansile lytic lesion in the third molar–ascending ramus of the mandible, with multiloculation (80%), resorbed teeth, and thinned cortical margins, describes most ameloblastomas. Unfortunately, odontogenic keratocysts, aneurysmal bone cysts, and giant cell tumors may also appear similarly. Ameloblastomas of the maxilla are usually centered in the premolar–first molar region and may grow into the maxillary sinus. On MRI mural nodules and high T1W intensity in cystic portions of the tumor and papillary projections are occasionally seen. Enhancement of nodules and septa is invariably present. The findings on enhanced MRI and the presence of mural nodules are unlikely in odontogenic keratocysts, aneurysmal bone cysts, and dentigerous cysts. However, there is still a tough differential between giant cell tumors and ameloblastomas. If the tumor is associated with an unerupted molar, go with ameloblastoma.

Unilocularity occurs in 20% of cases of ameloblastomas. These ameloblastomas are seen in a younger age group than those of the multilocular variety, and the recurrence rate (15%) of unilocular ameloblastomas is one fifth that of the multiloculated variety (75%). Unilocular ameloblastomas tend to occur around the third mandibular molar.

Notes

CASE 134

Aberrant Internal Carotid Artery

1. The inferior tympanic artery.

2. Glomus tympanicum.

3. A vascular intratympanic mass, hearing loss, and/or a bruit.

4. Objective. (The doc can hear it too.)

Reference

Sinnreich AI, Parisier SC, Cohen NL, Berreby M: Arterial malformations of the middle ear, *Otolaryngol Head Neck Surg* 92:194-206, 1984.

Cross-Reference

Neuroradiology: THE REQUISITES, pp 54-57.

Comment

For some reason, women are more likely to have aberrant carotid arteries, and the right side is affected more commonly than the left. Patients present with tinnitus and conductive hearing loss. Most surgeons avoid attempting to treat this source of tinnitus. High resolution CT is the study of choice for this anomaly. With an aberrant carotid artery, look for (1) enlargement of the inferior tympanic canaliculus seen anterolateral to the jugular bulb and posterolateral to the expected location of the carotid canal, (2) dehiscence along the posterolateral carotid canal, and (3) a soft tissue mass extending onto or near the cochlear promontory.

The fetal petrous carotid artery gives rise to the hyoid artery, which in turn gives rise to the stapedial artery that passes through the middle ear and gives rise to the middle meningeal artery. If the stapedial artery fails to regress it takes over the middle meningeal artery's supply, and the foramen spinosum does not develop. The hyoid artery should become the petrous carotid's caroticotympanic branch. If it does not regress it can anastomose with the inferior tympanic arterial branch of the ascending pharyngeal artery and take over the distal carotid artery's circulation. There are four middle ear vascular variants: (1) a persistent stapedial artery, (2) an aberrant course of the internal carotid artery, (3) an aberrant course of the internal carotid artery with a persistent stapedial artery, and (4) a pharyngosta-pedial artery.

Notes

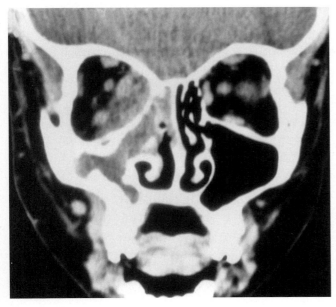

1. What is the most common cause of orbital cellulitis?

2. What is the vital structure that separates periorbital from orbital cellulitis?

3. How does disease spread from the sinuses to the orbits?

4. Infection in which sinus is least likely to cause orbital cellulitis?

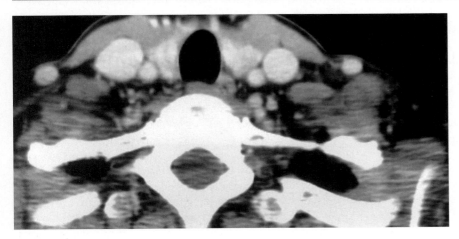

1. Put the following in order: roots, cords, peripheral nerves, divisions, trunks.

2. With what vessel does the brachial plexus have its most intimate association?

3. What percentage of patients with brachial plexopathies have trauma as the cause?

4. What are the most likely nontraumatic causes of brachial plexopathy?

CASE 135

Orbital Cellulitis
1. Spread from the paranasal sinuses (76%).
2. The orbital septum.
3. Via dehiscent bone, valveless veins, or ethmoidal penetrating arteries.
4. Maxillary sinus. When patients are erect or supine, the fluid remains dependent and well away from the orbit.

Reference
Weber AL, Mikulis DK: Inflammatory disorders of the paraorbital sinuses and their complications, *Radiol Clin North Am* 25:615-630, 1987.

Cross-Reference
Neuroradiology: THE REQUISITES, p 299.

Comment
Other causes of orbital cellulitis include trauma, penetrating injuries, dacryocystitis, and postsurgical and dermatologic infections. The danger of orbital cellulitis is that it can spread to the globe, optic nerve, cavernous sinus, meninges, and brain—leading to blindness, meningitis, epidural or cerebral abscess, thrombophlebitis, and phthisis bulbi. Drainage of the sinus or of subperiosteal, epidural, or intraconal abscesses may be required. Staphylococci and streptococci are the most common microorganisms cultured.

Once you see stranding of the intraconal fat in a patient with a fever and a proptotic, painful eye, call the clinician. Although it may just be edema in the fat from congestion, it behooves the physician to treat the patient with aggressive antibiotics and drainage if necessary. Periorbital or preseptal cellulitis is much more common than postseptal orbital cellulitis and is less disconcerting than when septum has been violated. Because the periorbita is such a good barrier to disease, it is not uncommon to see subperiosteal abscesses without conal or intraconal spread. CT is ideally suited to see the sinuses, the bone, the areas of dehiscence, and the potential dangers for the surgeon who has to treat the infection.

One of the more virulent infections is fulminant mucormycosis, which invariably necessitates orbital exenteration for cure. Otherwise, intracranial spread of mycotic infections may render the patient neurologically impaired. Spread appears to occur along blood vessels (arteries or veins) from the cavernous sinus. Emboli, vasculitis, and aneurysms may be deadly complications.

Notes

CASE 136

Brachial Plexus Schwannoma
1. Roots, trunks, divisions, cords, peripheral nerves.
2. The subclavian artery. The plexus runs superoposterior to the subclavian artery.
3. Approximately 50%.
4. Neoplasms (meningiomas, schwannomas, hemangiomas, sarcomas, metastatic disease, and lung cancers growing superiorly via a Pancoast tumor), lymphadenopathy, radiation damage, hygromas, and cervical ribs.

Reference
Iyer RB, Fenstermacher MJ, Libschitz HI: MR imaging of the treated brachial plexus, *AJR Am J Roentgenol* 167:225-229, 1996.

Cross-Reference
Neuroradiology: THE REQUISITES, p 437.

Comment
MRI in the sagittal plane is a good way to evaluate the cervical cord and brachial plexus all in one shot—it puts the plexus in cross section and allows display of the relationships with vessels very nicely. Remember that the plexus runs anterior to the middle and posterior scalene muscles and behind the anterior scalene muscle in the neck.

The brachial plexus is one of the dominant structures of the infrahyoid posterolateral/muscular space. Inflammatory lesions (resulting from virus, radiation, or spread from subclavian/jugular thrombophlebitis) may occur here, and traumatic injuries of the brachial plexus (Erb's palsy in the infant) may cause a brachial plexopathy. Malignancies of the brachial plexus include lymphadenopathy secondary to a head and neck primary tumor, lymphoma, chest primary tumor, or breast primary tumor. The hardest part of brachial plexus imaging is trying to distinguish radiation fibrosis, treated "dead nodes," and viable breast cancer lymph nodes. Treated nodes and scar tissue are dark on T2W scans—if you see something bright and avidly enhancing, suggest recurrent disease. All three may cause a brachial plexopathy. Paclitaxel (Taxol), a treatment for breast cancer, may cause a peripheral neuropathy that simulates brachial plexopathy.

Instrumentation and surgery in the region may also cause symptoms. Pancoast tumors may also elicit a Horner's syndrome. A Horner's syndrome may occur secondary to lesions anywhere along the sympathetic nervous system plexus in the neck, the hypothalamus of the brain, or the superior cervical ganglion region around the C7-T1 region.

Notes

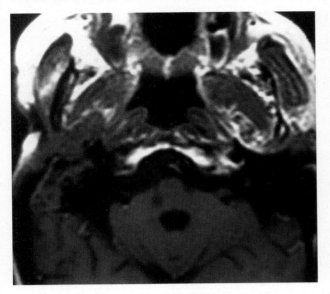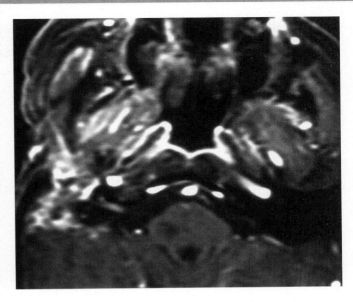

1. What are the most common malignancies to affect the external auditory canal?

2. Which has a more benign course, basal cell carcinoma or squamous cell carcinoma of the skin?

3. What is the effect on prognosis if an external auditory canal cancer spreads to the middle ear?

4. What two inflammatory conditions mimic external auditory canal malignancies?

CASE 138

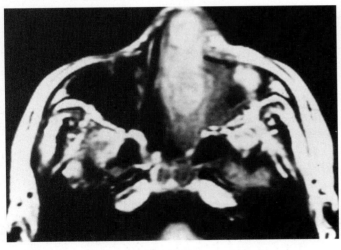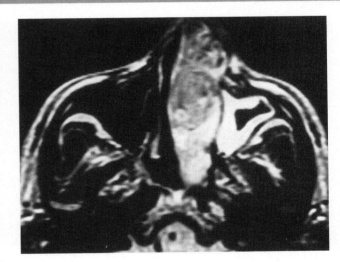

1. Why are some melanomas bright and some not on T1W scans?

2. Where in the sinonasal cavity are these lesions most common?

3. How often are they amelanotic?

4. What is the most common site of head and neck melanomas?

Skin Cancer Growing into the Ear

1. In adults (from most to least common), squamous cell carcinomas, basal cell carcinomas, and melanomas from adjacent skin. In children, rhabdomyosarcomas.

2. Basal cell carcinoma.

3. The 5-year survival rate decreases by 50%.

4. Malignant otitis externa and eosinophilic granuloma.

Reference

Pensak ML, Gleich LL, Gluckman JL, Shumrick KA: Temporal bone carcinoma: contemporary perspectives in the skull base surgical era, *Laryngoscope* 106:1234-1237, 1996.

Cross-Reference

Neuroradiology: THE REQUISITES, p 338.

Comment

Temporal bone malignancies are very difficult to eradicate once they have violated the middle ear and mastoid cavity. Grading of these ear tumors reflects their extent: Grade I—single site less than or equal to 1 cm; Grade II—single site greater than 1 cm; Grade III—transannular tumor extension; Grade IV—mastoid or petrous air cell invasion; Grade V—periauricular or contiguous extratemporal spread; and Grade VI—neck adenopathy, distant metastases, and infratemporal fossa invasion. Most are squamous cell carcinomas, but basal cell carcinomas and adenoid cystic carcinomas also occur in the temporal bone and ear. The latter two cancers have a much more benign course than squamous cell carcinoma. One of the critical determinants for taking an operative approach is how far medially the tumor goes—if the tumor stays lateral to the bony-cartilaginous external auditory canal, local resection is possible. Extension medially to the tympanic membrane necessitates more rigorous attention to the facial nerve, carotid artery, jugular vein, dura, and other essential structures. Radiation therapy is commonly required postoperatively. Clinical findings are otalgia, an aural mass, and an aural discharge.

In this case note the retraction of the skin and soft tissue posterior to the mandible, the infiltration of the parotid tissue, and the opacification of the temporal bone in the figure on the left. This tissue enhances in a solid fashion, unlike what one would expect with inflammatory disease of the mastoid air cells. I am not sure that I would pass the marrow signal of the right mandible as normal—the fat seems replaced.

Notes

Sinonasal Melanoma

1. Because the signal intensity varies depending on whether the melanoma is melanotic or amelanotic, on the amount of melanin present, and on the presence of intratumoral hemorrhage.

2. In the nasal compartment (with the anterior nasal septum and turbinates the preferred sites).

3. One third of the time.

4. The skin.

Reference

Yousem DM, Li C, Montone KT, Montgomery L, Loevner LA, Rao V, Chung TS, Kimura Y, Hayden RE, Weinstein GS: Primary malignant melanoma of the sinonasal cavity: MR imaging evaluation, *Radiographics* 16:1101-1110, 1996.

Cross-Reference

Neuroradiology: THE REQUISITES, pp 372-373.

Comment

Sinonasal melanoma, like ocular melanoma, is one of the few diagnoses one can pin down nicely with MRI on the basis of signal intensity characteristics. There are not too many well-defined or even ill-defined masses of the sinonasal cavity that are going to be relatively high in signal intensity on T1W MRI. The whole cavity may be studded with melanosis (I have also seen this in the oral cavity and oropharynx), making treatment difficult. Overall, patients with melanomas that have escaped the primary site fare pretty poorly.

Less than 1% of all melanomas occur in the sinonasal cavity, and usually they favor the nasal cavity (anterior nasal septum, lateral nasal wall, and inferior turbinates) over the paranasal sinuses (maxillary sinus most common). Complaints include nasal bleeding, nasal airway obstruction, deformity of the nose, hyposmia, facial pain, and visual disturbance. The peak incidence is in the fifth to seventh decades of life. Men are more commonly affected than women, and the prognosis is poor, with median survival times of 24 months.

Notes

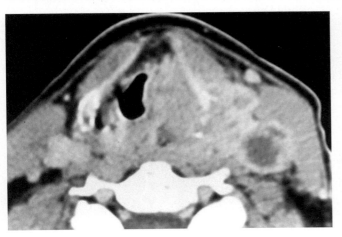
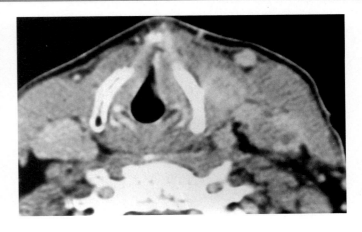

1. Which has a higher false positive rate for suggesting cartilage invasion by cancer, MRI or CT?

2. For which cartilage is imaging least accurate in predicting invasion, and why?

3. When does cartilage invasion preclude radiation therapy as a primary modality for treatment?

4. Which imaging finding has the lowest rate of false positive studies for cartilage invasion?

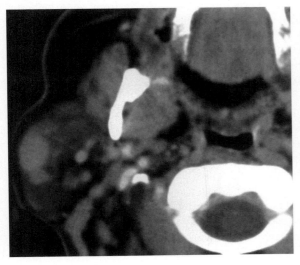
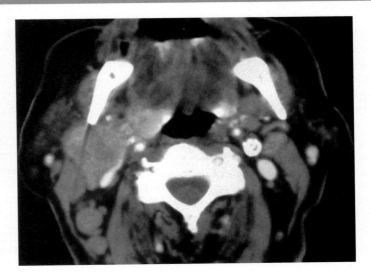

1. What are the most common causes of lymphadenopathy of the parotid gland?

2. Define Kimura's disease.

3. How often does sarcoidosis affect the parotid glands?

4. Why do Warthin's tumors only occur in the parotid glands and not in other salivary glands?

Cartilage Destruction by Hypopharyngeal Squamous Cell Carcinoma, Nodes, Paraglottic Spread

1. MRI.

2. The thyroid cartilage has a very high rate of false positive studies because of the potential for inflammatory reaction in the cartilage and because of its irregular ossification and chondrification.

3. Except in very limited, non–through and through invasion, radiotherapy is contraindicated with cartilage invasion.

4. Tumor crossing cartilage and growing into the strap muscles.

Reference

Zbaren P, Becker M, Lang H: Pretherapeutic staging of laryngeal carcinoma: clinical findings, computed tomography, and magnetic resonance imaging compared with histopathology, *Cancer* 77:1263-1273, 1996.

Cross-Reference

Neuroradiology: THE REQUISITES, pp 394-401.

Comment

You would think that radiologists would do pretty well in evaluating the laryngeal cartilages for invasion. It turns out that the perichondrium can react in an inflammatory way, leading to edema and inflammation within the cartilage that may simulate cancerous invasion. This can be manifest as sclerosis or erosion on CT and abnormal signal intensity and enhancement on MRI. The thyroid cartilage is particularly troublesome, with false positive studies in as many as 40% of patients with adjacent laryngeal cancer. Imaging is more accurate with the cricoid and arytenoid cartilages. On CT, try to identify focal erosions, sclerosis, and invasion into the strap muscles as your best criteria. For MRI, high signal intensity on T2W fat-suppressed scans in the cartilage, enhancement, and invasion into the strap muscles are most reliable. Unfortunately, sometimes a voice box is taken out for suspicious imaging findings when there is no cancer. Tragic. The alternative is to perform elegant voice conservation surgery but leave tumor behind in a cartilage or to assign a patient to a radiation treatment that is ineffective against the tumor.

Cartilage invasion is also seen in 26% to 50% of hypopharyngeal carcinomas. The thyroid cartilage is most commonly affected.

Notes

Lymph Nodes in the Parotid Gland

1. Drainage of infections and superficial cancers around the ear and scalp, HIV, sarcoidosis, and lymphoma.

2. A disease in which the salivary glands and lymph nodes show focal tumoral lesions with vascular proliferation and eosinophilia.

3. In 10% to 30% of cases (usually bilaterally).

4. Because of the late encapsulation of the parotid gland embryologically, it is the only salivary gland to incorporate lymphoid tissue within it. Warthin's tumors are of lymphatic origin.

Reference

Gollub MJ, Gruen DR, Dershaw DD: Merkel cell carcinoma: CT findings in 12 patients, *AJR Am J Roentgenol* 167:617-620, 1996.

Cross-Reference

Neuroradiology: THE REQUISITES, pp 403-408.

Comment

The histologic diagnosis in this case was Merkel cell carcinoma. Merkel cell carcinoma is a skin cancer that presents with a violaceous subcutaneous mass arising from neuroendocrine (tactile neurosensors) cells in the basal epidermis. Recurrences (25% to 77%), lymph node metastases (31% to 83%), and hematogenous metastases (33% to 50%) occur frequently. On CT, the primary tumors and their nodal metastases are said to be hyperdense to muscle. The head and neck is the most common site of these tumors. Do not forget—if asked what is the most common primary site of a head and neck cancer, say the skin!

Kimura's disease is a disease with salivary gland and lymph node manifestations seen in the male (4 times greater than female) Asian population. One sees nodes in the neck and parotid glands that are enlarged and enhance dramatically. Eosinophilia may be present in the blood stream. Kikuchi-Fujimoto disease (subacute necrotizing histiocytic lymphadenitis) also presents with cervical adenopathy and fever and usually spontaneously resolves; however, because patients are at risk for developing systemic lupus erythematosus, many people believe this to be an autoimmune disorder. Women are affected more than men.

Notes

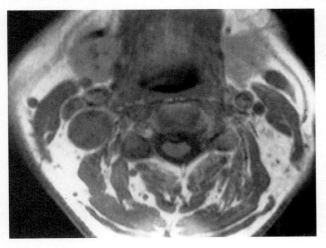 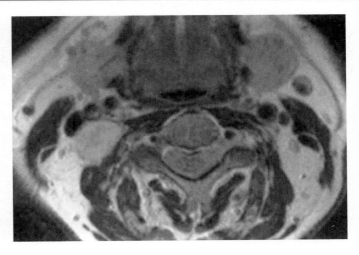

1. What are the two sources of carotid space schwannomas?

2. How can one distinguish a vagal schwannoma from a sympathetic plexus schwannoma?

3. What is the mechanism of cystic accumulation in schwannomas?

4. What percentage of schwannomas occur in the head and neck?

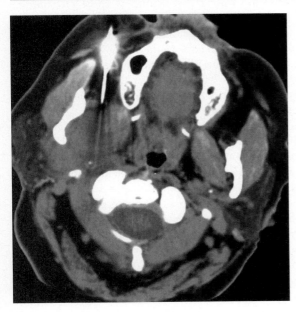

1. How is the parapharyngeal space subdivided?

2. What are the two most common tumors of the prestyloid and poststyloid parapharyngeal spaces?

3. What is the best way to distinguish a paraganglioma from a schwannoma or meningioma?

4. What happens to the carotid artery with a prestyloid parapharyngeal space mass?

Cervical Sympathetic Plexus Schwannoma

1. The vagus nerve and sympathetic plexus fibers.

2. Vagal schwannomas tend to splay the carotid artery and jugular vein apart, whereas sympathetic plexus schwannomas usually push both forward.

3. It may be from mucinous degeneration, microcystic elements, hemorrhagic by-products, hyperproteinaceous debris, or central necrosis owing to outstripping of blood supply.

4. Twenty-five percent to 45%.

Reference

Catalano P, Fang-Hui E, Som PM: Fluid-fluid levels in benign neurogenic tumors, *AJNR Am J Neuroradiol* 18:385-387, 1997.

Cross-Reference

Neuroradiology: THE REQUISITES, pp 432-437.

Comment

The superior cervical ganglion resides opposite the second and third vertebras. It lies between the carotid sheath and the longus capitis muscle. Fibers connect to cranial nerves IX through XII and the hypothalamus via the cavernous sinus and to the middle cervical ganglion. The middle cervical ganglion is variably present and, when found, is located near the sixth cervical vertebra near the inferior thyroid artery. Branches run behind the carotid artery and along the trachea. The lowermost cervical sympathetic ganglion is the stellate ganglion (inferior cervical or cervicothoracic ganglion), which lies anterior and lateral to the longus colli muscle at the C7-T1 level adjacent to the first thoracic rib. A Horner's syndrome may be due to lesions all along this pathway. If the patient has a lung apex mass and a Horner's syndrome, be suspicious of a Pancoast tumor eroding through the chest wall to affect the stellate ganglion. Carotid dissections, as causes of Horner's syndrome, usually affect the sympathetic plexus more superiorly.

Notes

Pleomorphic Adenoma of the Deep Lobe of the Parotid Gland

1. Into the prestyloid and poststyloid (carotid space) parapharyngeal spaces.

2. Squamous cell carcinoma (from the mucosa) and pleomorphic adenoma (from ectopic salivary rests or deep lobe parotid masses) for the prestyloid parapharyngeal space, and schwannomas and paragangliomas for the poststyloid parapharyngeal space.

3. Dynamic enhanced imaging, plotting the early downward spike of a paraganglioma.

4. It is displaced posteriorly, if at all.

Reference

Yousem DM, Sack MJ, Weinstein GS, Hayden RE: Computed tomography–guided aspirations of parapharyngeal and skull base masses, *Skull Base Surg* 5:131-136, 1995.

Cross-Reference

Neuroradiology: THE REQUISITES, pp 385-386, 419-420, 424.

Comment

The usual issue with a parapharyngeal space pleomorphic adenoma is, "Does it arise from ectopic minor salivary gland rests in the parapharyngeal space, or is it growing off the deep lobe of the parotid gland?" If the lesion is large, which it frequently is because this is a clinically occult zone, the question may be particularly hard to answer. Attempt to find the parapharyngeal fat. If it is displaced anteromedially, you have your answer—it is a deep lobe parotid mass. If the fat surrounds the lesion or caps it, it is most likely from the parapharyngeal space. If the lesion widens the stylomandibular tunnel, it is most likely of parotid origin. These points are not exactly moot. Surgeons describe how easy and how much fun it is to "deliver" a parapharyngeal space pleomorphic adenoma—they just reach up with a finger from a submandibular approach, dissect around with a forefinger, grab above the lesion, and pull it out. Deep lobe parotid masses are much more difficult to remove, and the facial nerve becomes much more of an issue.

Because this lesion has a tail of tissue that buds medially to the ramus of the mandible and widens the distance from mandible to styloid process, I believe it arises from the deep lobe of the parotid gland. Strangely enough, the patient refused surgery after my beautiful CT-guided aspiration, so we can debate this case forever. I guess I scared her off.

Notes

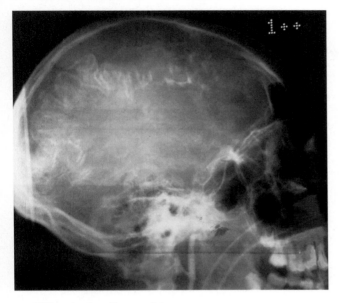

1. What is the diagnosis?

2. Define the clinical triad of Sturge-Weber syndrome.

3. What is the histology of the facial and intracranial lesion?

4. Define Dyke-Davidoff-Masson syndrome.

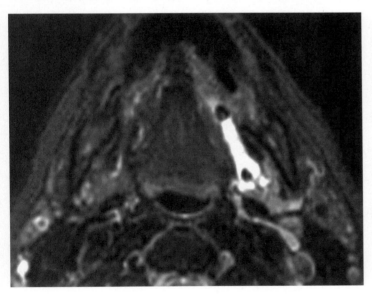 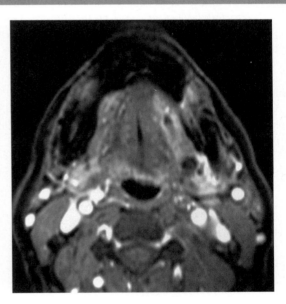

1. How often do patients with calculi in their submandibular glands present with painless masses?

2. For a painful submandibular mass, what study should be ordered?

3. How often is a painful submandibular mass the result of calculus disease?

4. What percentage of salivary gland masses are in the submandibular gland?

Sturge-Weber Syndrome

1. Sturge-Weber syndrome, or encephalotrigeminal angiomatosis.

2. Seizures (75% to 90%), mental retardation (50%), and port-wine nevus of the face (90%).

3. A vascular malformation of the first division of the fifth cranial nerve in the face and the venous capillary plexus of the brain.

4. Brain hemiatrophy with calvarial thickening, and sinus enlargement ipsilateral to the atrophy.

Reference

Benedikt RA, Brown DC, Walker R, Ghaed VN, Mitchell M, Geyer CA: Sturge-Weber syndrome: cranial MR imaging with GD-DTPA, *AJNR Am J Neuroradiol* 14:409-415, 1993.

Cross-Reference

Neuroradiology: THE REQUISITES, pp 270-271.

Comment

The port-wine stain of Sturge-Weber syndrome is thought to be a capillary hemangioma, the so-called nevus flammeus. The patients may also have glaucoma, buphthalmos, hemiparesis, and hemianopsia, depending on what part of the cerebrum is involved. A leptomeningeal angioma is present in association with anomalous venous drainage of the brain (absent cortical veins). One may also see an enlarged choroidal plexus owing to either anomalous venous drainage or an angioma. Gyriform enhancement of the cortex is probably due to the overlying leptomeningeal abnormality. Reduced arterial flow is present. If Sturge-Weber syndrome affects both hemispheres, the IQ is affected more severely. Hypermyelination may be present in the white matter.

Glaucoma can occur with Sturge-Weber syndrome, Klippel-Trénaunay-Weber syndrome, and oculodermal melanocytosis—three uncommon neural crest disorders.

The calcification seen on this plain film is in middle layers of the cortex underlying the leptomeningeal vascular malformation on the surface of the brain. The calcification may be seen to progress posteriorly to anteriorly with time.

William Allen Sturge (1850-1919) and Frederick Parkes Weber (1863-1962) were British physicians.

Notes

Submandibular Gland Calculus on MRI

1. One third of the time.

2. CT (because MRI is insensitive to calculi detection).

3. As high as 80% of the time.

4. Ten percent.

Reference

Kaneda T, Minami M, Ozawa K, Akimoto Y, Kawana T, Okada H, Yamamoto H, Suzuki H, Sasaki Y: MR of the submandibular gland: normal and pathologic states, *AJNR Am J Neuroradiol* 17:1575-1581, 1996.

Cross-Reference

Neuroradiology: THE REQUISITES, p 415.

Comment

Yes, occasionally you find a calculus on MRI, but I would not recommend using this modality as the primary means to evaluate patients for sialolithiasis. People have been experimenting with MR sialography and have obtained reasonable pictures of the ductal system, but I would reserve those studies to replace sialography, not to replace CT for detecting stones. In too many cases the stone may be very tiny and lodged just at the orifice of the duct. In this far distal location, air (outside the duct, or for that matter within the duct) on MRI may look just like a calcified stone. I believe in CT. There are very few calculi that are not radiopaque on CT.

Notes

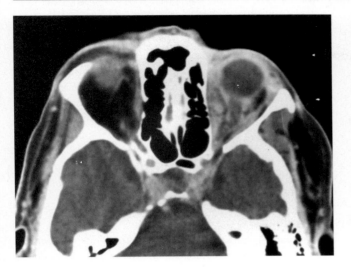
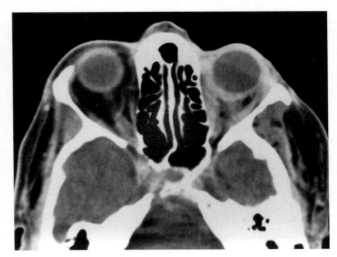

1. What is the histology of this lesion, and how does one know?

2. Are most metastases to the orbit intra- or extraconal?

3. What bone lining the orbit is most commonly affected by a metastasis?

4. Are ocular metastases common?

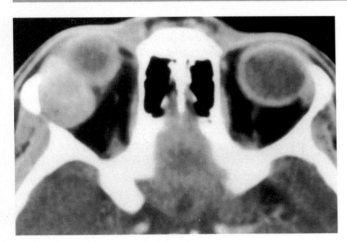

1. Name the three groupings of lacrimal fossa masses.

2. In what percentage of orbital pseudotumor cases is the lacrimal gland involved?

3. Is remodeling of the bone a good sign to suggest benignity in lacrimal gland tumors?

4. What nonlacrimal gland lesions may enlarge the lacrimal fossa?

CASE 145

Breast Carcinoma Metastasis to the Orbit

1. Scirrhous carcinoma from a breast primary. One knows this because there is enophthalmos associated with a large amount of tumor burden.

2. Extraconal.

3. The greater wing of the sphenoid.

4. Yes, very common, but they do not present clinically.

Reference
Gunalp T, Gunduz K: Metastatic orbital tumors, *Jpn J Ophthalmopathy* 39:65-70, 1995.

Cross-Reference
Neuroradiology: THE REQUISITES, pp 284, 287.

Comment
Metastases to the globe tend to occur in the uveal tract or the retina, whereas extraocular metastases are usually to the bones around the orbit. Presentations include proptosis, blurred vision, and motility deficits. The most common primary tumors to go to the orbit are neuroblastomas (children) and tumors of the breast, lung, thyroid, prostate, and kidney. Orbital symptoms may precede the detection of the primary tumor in about 25% to 33% of cases. When orbital metastases occur, the prognosis is pretty poor (14% 5-year survival). The differential diagnosis of an infiltrating intraconal mass includes lymphoma and pseudotumor. Less likely possibilities are plexiform neurofibroma and arteriovenous malformation.

In adults, *ocular* metastases account for 90% of *orbital* metastases. Spread is usually hematogenous. Looking at random eye bank donations, ocular metastases occur in about 1% of individuals. Patients with carcinoma who donate their eyes display macroscopic evidence of ocular metastases in 4.7% of cases. Histopathologically, 12.6% of patients with carcinoma who donate their eyes show ocular metastases. Leukemia, which once accounted for a high percentage of ocular metastases, is being better treated, so noncarcinomatous ocular metastases are decreasing.

Notes

CASE 146

Lacrimal Gland Mass—Adenoid Cystic Carcinoma

1. Salivary gland epithelial tumors (pleomorphic adenoma, adenoid cystic carcinoma, malignant mixed tumors, mucoepidermoid carcinomas, adenocarcinoma), germ cell tumors (dermoids), and lymphoid lesions (lymphoma, sarcoid, pseudotumor, Wegener's granulomatosis).

2. Fifteen percent.

3. Actually, no!

4. Dermoids, schwannomas, myxomas, hematic cysts, and granulomas.

Reference
Vangveeravong S, Katz SE, Rootman J, White V: Tumors arising in the palpebral lobe of the lacrimal gland, *Ophthalmology* 103:1606-1612, 1996.

Cross-Reference
Neuroradiology: THE REQUISITES, p 300.

Comment
The lacrimal gland is similar to the parotid gland in that it can have tumors of "salivary gland" origin and lymphoproliferative diseases. The two glands may share the same diseases, including sarcoidosis, Sjögren's syndrome, Wegener's granulomatosis, Mikulicz's disease, lymphoma, pleomorphic adenomas (most common benign tumor), and adenoid cystic carcinomas (most common malignant tumor). In addition, the lacrimal fossa may be the site of the epidermoid-dermoid line of lesions. In contrast, lacrimal sac tumors (on the other side of the orbit) are often of epithelial origin, such as squamous cell carcinomas or transitional cell carcinomas. Mucoepidermoid carcinoma is the most common minor salivary gland tumor to affect the lacrimal sac.

More than half of patients with lymphoma in their lacrimal glands have it as a manifestation of systemic disease, usually NHL. This contrasts with lymphoma of the conjunctiva, which is usually localized to that site. The lacrimal fossa is the most common site of lymphoma in the orbit.

Notes

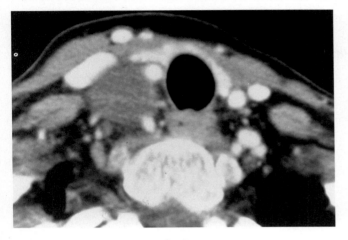 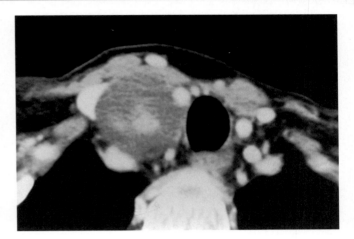

1. What is the pertinent finding?
2. Is the lesion thyroidal or extrathyroidal?
3. In what space in the neck is the lesion?
4. What does the differential diagnosis include?

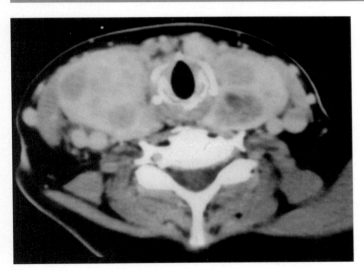

1. What is the most commonly detected primary tumor to metastasize to the thyroid gland?
2. What are the most common primary tumors to metastasize to the thyroid gland?
3. What is the most common primary tumor to metastasize to the sinonasal cavity?
4. What does the differential diagnosis of multiple masses in the thyroid gland include?

CASE 147

Vagal Schwannoma

1. Cystic-solid mass in the lateral neck.

2. Extrathyroidal.

3. The infrahyoid carotid space.

4. Schwannoma, extrathyroidal goitrous tissue, nodal metastases, and lymphangioma.

Reference

Som PM, Braun IF, Shapiro MD, Reede DL, Curtin HD, Zimmerman RA: Tumors of the parapharyngeal space and upper neck: MR imaging characteristics, *Radiology* 164:823-829, 1987.

Cross-Reference

Neuroradiology: THE REQUISITES, p 432.

Comment

The majority of carotid space masses are benign. Of these, two classic lesions are the vagus schwannoma and the paraganglioma. Situated posterior to the carotid artery, vagus nerve lesions tend to displace the carotid artery anteriorly, and splay the carotid and jugular vessels. Schwannomas of the vagus nerve are usually well-defined, rounded structures that are hypodense to muscle on CT and that enhance moderately. The lesions are well demarcated on T1W imaging owing to the high signal intensity fat around the carotid sheath and around the parapharyngeal space. Whereas on an enhanced CT the border between the schwannoma and carotid artery or jugular vein may be indistinguishable, on MR it is possible to identify the flow voids of the carotid artery and jugular vein from the enhancing solid tumor. Occasionally schwannomas may be cystic and will demonstrate characteristic density and intensity features for cyst fluid. Schwannomas also may hemorrhage within themselves.

Notes

CASE 148

Renal Cell Carcinoma Metastasis to Thyroid Gland

1. Renal cell carcinoma.

2. Lung and breast tumors. (But they are often clinically silent and only found at autopsy.)

3. Renal cell carcinoma.

4. Lymphoma, goiter, metastases, thyroiditis, cysts, and multiple primary tumors.

Reference

Haugen BR, Nawaz S, Cohn A, Shroyer K, Burn PA Jr, Liechty DR, Ridgway EC: Secondary malignancy of the thyroid gland: a case report and review of the literature, *Thyroid* 4:297-300, 1994.

Cross-Reference

Neuroradiology: THE REQUISITES, pp 440-441.

Comment

Although renal cell carcinoma is the classic metastasis to go to the thyroid gland, when one includes perithyroid lesions, lung cancer turns out to be numero uno. Only 25% of patients presenting with metastases to the thyroid gland have a known primary tumor at the time of fine needle aspiration. Because clear cell carcinomas may occur in tumors of both kidney and thyroid origin, it is important for the pathologist to perform immunohistochemical stains for colloid or thyroglobulin to determine the origin of these lesions. A positive oil red O stain for fat suggests renal origin. When a patient has bilateral masses in the thyroid gland, a multinodular goiter, lymphoma, multifocal thyroid cancer, unusual thyroiditis, and metastases should come to mind.

The first manifestation of kidney cancer may be from a head and neck metastasis.

Notes

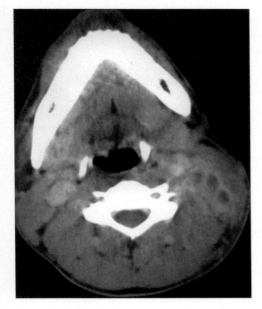

1. What are the typical findings on CT of tuberculous lymphadenitis?

2. What organism is most commonly cultured from tuberculous adenitis?

3. What percentage of extrapulmonary tuberculosis cases are manifest as cervical adenitis?

4. What is the treatment of choice for tuberculous adenitis?

CASE 150

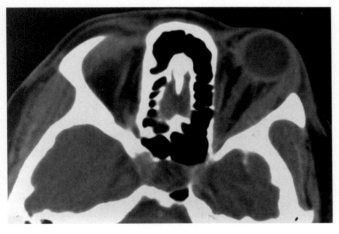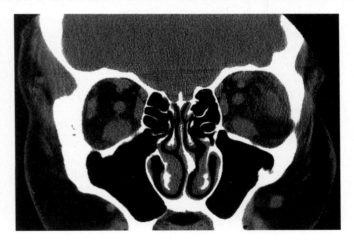

1. What structures of the orbit may be affected by pseudotumor?

2. To what is pseudotumor exquisitely sensitive?

3. What does pseudotumor look like on T2W MRI?

4. What are the classic three diagnoses of the orbit that go together with most differentials?

Tuberculous Adenitis

1. Conglomerate masses with irregular enhancement, with diffuse infiltration of adjacent muscle and fat. Often there are large, dense masses with rim enhancement. Calcified nodes may also be present.

2. *Mycobacterium bovis.*

3. Fifteen percent.

4. Excision or triple drug therapy.

Reference

Moon WK, Han MH, Chang KH, Im J-G, Kim H-J, Sung KJ, Lee HK: CT and MR imaging of head and neck tuberculosis, *Radiographics* 17:391-402, 1997.

Cross-Reference

Neuroradiology: THE REQUISITES, pp 405-406.

Comment

Patients with tuberculous adenitis present most commonly without constitutional signs, but with just a firm, painless neck mass. Pulmonary tuberculosis may or may not be evident at the time of presentation (some say ongoing pulmonary tuberculosis or a history of it can be elicited in 50% of patients, and 100% are PPD positive). Reede and Bergeron describe four patterns of disease: (1) multichambered, thick-walled nodal masses with ring enhancement and preserved adjacent fascial planes; (2) a large necrotic mass with thick walls and adjacent fascial infiltration and fatty stranding (the cold abscess); (3) a homogeneous nodal mass with or without enhancement, but with no necrosis and no infiltration; and (4) a nodal mass with rim enhancement and no necrosis, but with infiltration into adjacent areas. The most common and distinctive pattern is the multichambered one, with necrosis usually seen in the posterior triangle of the neck. Bilateral or unilateral adenopathy may be present. Ninety percent of cases of extrapulmonary tuberculosis in the head and neck occur in lymph nodes. In descending order, the larynx, temporal bone, pharynx, sinonasal cavity, orbit, and skull base are the next most common sites of disease.

Differential diagnosis? Metastatic nodes, any necrotizing cervical adenitis, Kikuchi's disease, and lymphoma.

Notes

Orbital Pseudotumor

1. You name it—every part of the orbit from lid to nerve may be affected.

2. Steroids.

3. It is intermediate to low in intensity.

4. Pseudotumor, lymphoma, and sarcoid.

Reference

Bencherif B, Zouaoui A, Chedid G, Kujas M, Van Effenterre R, Marsault C: Intracranial extension of an idiopathic orbital inflammatory pseudotumor, *AJNR Am J Neuroradiol* 14:181-184, 1994.

Cross-Reference

Neuroradiology: THE REQUISITES, p 297.

Comment

Idiopathic orbital inflammatory pseudotumor is a granulomatous inflammation of the orbit characterized by lots of giant cells, plasma cells, and lymphocytes on pathology. Chemosis, pain, and proptosis are common. The lacrimal gland is one of the most common structures of the orbit to be involved. If the cavernous sinus is primarily involved, producing a painful ophthalmoplegia, the disorder is called Tolosa-Hunt syndrome. With Tolosa-Hunt syndrome, orbital apex involvement is frequent. The symptoms are due to involvement of cranial nerves III to VI in the cavernous sinus.

Response to steroids is classic for pseudotumor, with over 75% showing an initial response and 37% cured by steroids. However, recurrence rates are high (52%) for areas of the orbit other than the optic nerve, in which cure rates are over 90% with steroids. The more bulky and fibrotic the pseudotumor mass, the lower the cure rate. All areas of the orbit, from lid to gland to muscle to nerve to sclera to conjunctiva to sac, may be affected with pseudotumor of the orbit. After making this statement in a previous case, I showed a case of superior ophthalmic vein enlargement to a resident in Montreal. She included pseudotumor in the differential diagnosis for the cause of superior ophthalmic vein enlargement. I had to retract my comment. Pseudotumor usually does not affect the arteries or veins unless the orbital apex is obstructed. Gallium scintigraphy is negative with pseudotumor but positive with lymphoma and sarcoidosis.

Notes

Challenge Cases

CASE 151

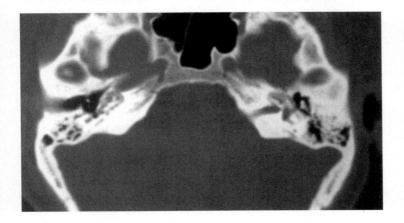 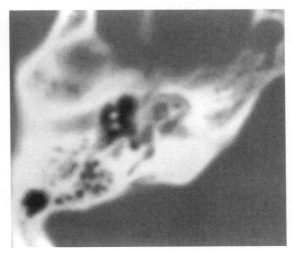

1. Describe the two classic sites of otospongiosis.

2. How does the disease manifest in these two sites?

3. What does the differential diagnosis of otospongiosis include?

4. Describe the stereotypical patient with otospongiosis, osteogenesis imperfecta, late stage Paget's disease, and syphilis.

CASE 152

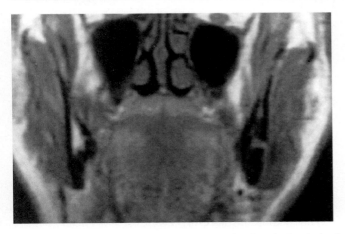 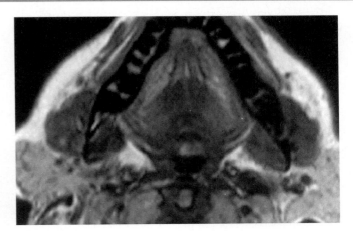

1. What are the most likely causes of a fistula leading from the skin into the mandible?

2. What does the differential diagnosis of mandibular marrow fat replacement on T1W scans include?

3. What is the significance of periosteal, cortical, and marrow invasion by neoplasm?

4. What important neural structure runs in the mandible?

Cochlear and Fenestral Otospongiosis

1. The oval window (anterior margin first) and the cochlea (basal turn first).

2. It is predominantly lytic around the cochlea in cochlear otospongiosis, but it manifests with lucent (or dense in the late phase) bone anterior to and narrowing the oval window with fenestral otospongiosis.

3. Osteogenesis imperfecta, very late stage Paget's disease, and otosyphilis.

4. Otospongiosis occurs most frequently in women in their 20s. Osteogenesis imperfecta is most common in children with brittle bones and blue sclera. Paget's disease occurs in the elderly. Ostosyphilis is usually seen in adults with systemic syphilitic infection.

Reference

Valvassori GE: Imaging of otosclerosis, *Otolaryngol Clin North Am* 26:359-371, 1993.

Cross-Reference

Neuroradiology: THE REQUISITES, p 351.

Comment

The term otosclerosis is a misnomer and the most confusing aspect of cochlear otospongiosis. Except in the very late stages of the disease and/or after therapy, this is a lytic process around the cochlea (like a halo). Eighty-five percent of cases of otospongiosis are of the fenestral type, most commonly visualized as decalcification of the margins of the oval window. Later, new bone may form along the anterior margin of the oval window. Fenestral otosclerosis converts to a more bone-forming appearance earlier than cochlear otosclerosis, effectively closing the oval window. At the oval window, the foot plate of the stapes can be affected, becoming fixed to the closed window and necessitating stapedectomy. Fixation of the stapes may lead to a conductive form of hearing loss. Fenestral otosclerosis is bilateral in approximately 85% of patients.

Cochlear otosclerosis is also called retrofenestral otosclerosis. Although conductive hearing loss is most commonly seen in cochlear otosclerosis, one may see sensorineural hearing loss as well. This may be due to compromise of the spiral ligament or toxic proteases that affect the nerve cells of the cochlea.

Although a few articles have described MRI features of otosclerosis (Saunders JE, Derebery MJ, Lo WW: Magnetic resonance imaging of otosclerosis, *Ann Otol Rhinol Laryngol* 104:826-829, 1995, for one), CT clearly is the mainstay of imaging for otospongiosis. It has been suggested that MRI with contrast shows active osteolysis with enhancement and can gauge activity of disease better than CT.

Notes

Perimandibular Fistula

1. Odontogenic infection, squamous cell carcinoma, Burkitt's lymphoma, and actinomycosis. Postoperative flap reconstruction with mandibular resection and postirradiation account for some iatrogenic cases.

2. Infection, neoplasm, traumatic edema, fibrosis, and radiation-induced osteonecrosis.

3. If the periosteum is invaded by tumor, surgeons perform a marginal corticectomy for surgical cure. If the periosteum is not involved, the periosteum is used as the margin for tumor resection. If the cortex is involved, a segmental mandibular resection is performed; however, this may not necessitate complete mandibular prosthetic replacement. If the marrow is infiltrated with tumor, a wide resection is required, often necessitating a graft or prosthetic mandibular surgery.

4. A branch of the mandibular nerve (inferior alveolar nerve) runs in the inferior alveolar canal and is a source of perineural spread of tumor.

Reference

Abrams JJ, Berger SB: Oral-maxillary sinus fistula (oroantral fistula): clinical features and findings on multiplanar CT, *AJR Am J Roentgenol* 165:1273-1276, 1995.

Cross-Reference

Neuroradiology: THE REQUISITES, pp 388-392.

Comment

Actinomyces israelii, a gram-positive branching anaerobic bacterium, is the classic organism to cause a cutaneous fistula from the mandible. This occurs in patients with poor dentition or dental abscesses and osteomyelitis. Extensive fibrosis associated with the lesion may lead to decreased T1W and T2W signal. It is an indolent infection associated with weight loss and low grade fever. Nodal disease is usually seen as well. Tumors rarely cause skin fistulas unless they are along a biopsy tract. Burkitt's lymphoma is associated with submandibular/mandibular disease and is associated with Epstein-Barr viral infection.

The findings of a defect in the cortex of the left mandible near a tooth and replacement of bright marrow fat on the T1W scan suggest, first and foremost, a dental extraction infection. This is far and away the most common thing to consider here, with carious dental disease number two. In this case, no dental manipulations had been performed. The information that there was a tract leading through the gingiva to the buccal mucosa and to the skin surface was provided by the otorhinolaryngologist. No neoplasm was found.

Notes

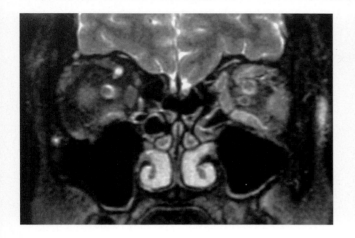
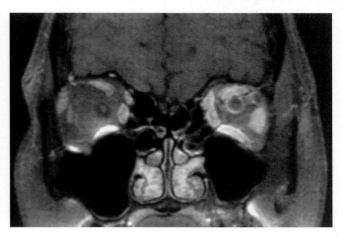

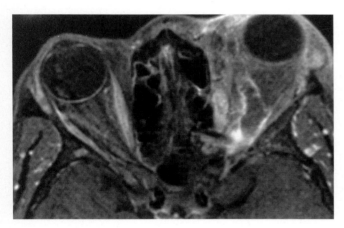

1. Given the muscular and vascular findings, what is the most likely diagnosis?

2. What are the most common causes of extraocular muscle enlargement unilaterally?

3. What are the causes of superior ophthalmic vein thrombosis or enlargement?

4. Differentiate between dural vascular malformations of the cavernous sinus and cavernous carotid artery fistulas.

Dural Arteriovenous Fistula with Superior Ophthalmic Vein Occlusion Causing Proptosis and Extraocular Muscle Enlargement

1. Dural fistula with superior ophthalmic vein thrombosis.

2. Thyroid eye disease, sinusitis with myositis, pseudotumor of the orbit, superior ophthalmic vein thrombosis, cavernous carotid fistulas, orbital cellulitis, lymphoma, rhabdomyosarcoma, and myxoma.

3. Dural arteriovenous malformations or fistulas, venous varices, and hypercoagulable states. Aspergillosis and mucormycosis infections also have a predilection for vascular thrombosis. Thyroid eye disease with orbital apex crowding may cause superior ophthalmic vein enlargement.

4. Cavernous carotid artery fistulas are usually single-hole, direct communications between the cavernous sinus in the carotid artery. They are usually traumatic in origin and are usually treated with balloon or coil embolotherapy. Dural vascular malformations are more common in women; they represent a true dural vascular fistula with a nidus and are treated with particulate therapy. They are less likely to occur as a result of trauma.

Reference

Cognard C, Gobin YP, Pierot L, Bailly AL, Houdart E, Casasco A, Chiras J, Merland JJ: Cerebral dural arteriovenous fistulas: clinical and angiographic correlation with a revised classification of venous drainage, *Radiology* 194:671-680, 1995.

Cross-Reference

Neuroradiology: THE REQUISITES, pp 496-498.

Comment

I like the new classification of intracranial dural AVFs proposed by Cognard and colleagues. Type I drains to a venous sinus with antegrade flow, type IIa to a venous sinus with retrograde filling of sinuses, type IIb to a venous sinus with retrograde flow into cortical veins, type III to cortical veins, type IV to cortical veins with venous ectasia, and type V to spinal dural veins. The rate of intracranial hypertension and hemorrhage increases from type I to type IV, and the presence of myelopathy is 50% in type V. After the transverse sinus, the cavernous sinus is the most common site of dural AVFs, but the course is much more benign than that of noncavernous fistulas with respect to intracranial complications. Most (>85%) cavernous sinus AVFs are type I by virtue of antegrade drainage to the sinus; rarely there is drainage to the sinus with retrograde filling of cortical veins.

Complications of cavernous carotid fistulas include ischemia of the optic nerves or dural thrombosis leading to intracranial high pressure and/or venous infarctions.

Notes

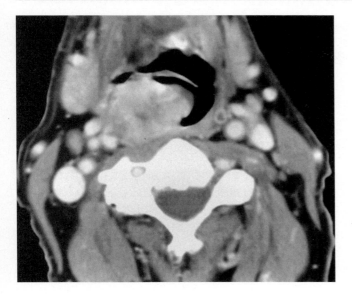

1. What is the most likely diagnosis of this lesion, which was thought to be submucosal at endoscopy?

2. What portion of the pharynx is involved with this lesion?

3. What are the common histologic diagnoses of non–squamous cell submucosal masses of the pharynx?

4. When dealing with hypopharyngeal masses, what are the critical determinants of spread?

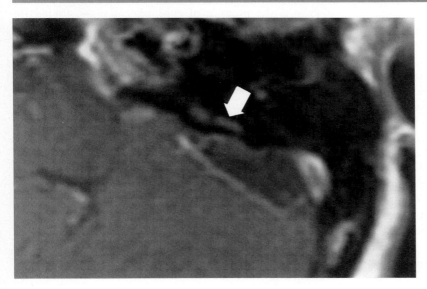

1. What structure is enhancing (shown by the arrow)?

2. What entities are associated with this structure's enhancement?

3. What malignancy of the endolymphatic sac occurs in this location?

4. What is the typical MRI picture of Meniere's disease?

Submucosal Aerodigestive System Mass—Malignant Fibrous Histiocytoma of the Posterior Pharynx

1. Squamous cell carcinoma—an occult mucosal focus of squamous cell carcinoma with deep submucosal spread is more commonly seen than primary non-squamous submucosal masses of the pharynx.

2. Because the lesion extends above the epiglottis, it encompasses the posterior pharyngeal wall of the oropharynx, and because it extends from the pharyngoepiglottic fold inferiorly, it also includes the hypopharynx.

3. Lymphoma, sarcomas, malignant fibrous histiocytomas (MFHs), rhabdomyo(sarco)mas, minor salivary gland tumors, and neurogenic tumors. Synovial sarcomas also occur here.

4. They frequently extend to and around the carotid artery. They may also spread into the prevertebral musculature. Both of these findings may lead to unresectable disease. They also invade the cartilage.

Reference

Murphey MD, Gross TM, Rosenthal HG: From the archives of the AFIP: musculoskeletal malignant fibrous histiocytoma—radiologic-pathologic correlation, *Radiographics* 14:807-826, 1994.

Cross-Reference

Neuroradiology: THE REQUISITES, pp 392-394, 428.

Comment

MFH is much more commonly seen as a soft tissue (rather than osseous) tumor of the extremities in an older individual. In fact, MFH accounts for 20% to 30% of all sarcomas of the soft tissues, but only 5% of the tumors occur in the head and neck. The soft tissues, orbit, and sinonasal cavities are the most common sites of MFH in the neck. It may develop in an area that was previously irradiated or in which surgery had been performed. The lesion is extraordinarily aggressive in the bones, a little less so in the soft tissues. It may have calcification visible on imaging in 5% to 20% of cases. The tumor may be well encapsulated in the head and neck, whereas elsewhere it tends to invade muscular compartments and neurovascular structures.

Of the MFHs I have seen, most show dark signal intensity on all MRI pulse sequences, presumably owing to the fibrous nature of the lesion. Angiomatoid fibrous histiocytomas often occur in the skin and subcutaneous tissues of the head and neck—they present in patients less than 20 years old.

Notes

Meniere's Disease

1. The vestibular aqueduct (endolymphatic sac).

2. Labyrinthitis, Meniere's disease, and perilymphatic fistulas.

3. Papillary adenomatoid carcinoma (low grade adenocarcinoma of endolymphatic sac origin).

4. A normal study.

Reference

Tanioka H, Kaga K, Zusho H, Araki T, Sasaki Y: MR of the endolymphatic duct and sac: findings in Meniere disease, *AJNR Am J Neuroradiol* 18:45-52, 1997.

Reference

Neuroradiology: THE REQUISITES, pp 352-353.

Comment

Many recent publications have focused on the ability of ultra-thin-section, high resolution, three-dimensional Fourier transform T2W gradient echo MRI scans to visualize the endolymphatic sac in normal individuals. By the same token, the sac may not be visualized in patients with Meniere's disease (endolymphatic hydrops), presumably because of fibrosis in and/or around the endolymphatic sac. Obstruction of the endolymphatic duct produces the symptoms of Meniere's disease—dizziness, vertigo, and tinnitus. Another finding reported anecdotally is the presence of enhancement in or around the endolymphatic duct, as demonstrated here. I am uncertain whether this truly represents a nearby vein or the duct itself, but in either case I "call it" when the history includes Meniere's disease.

Included in the differential diagnosis of Meniere's disease is chronic labyrinthitis and a labyrinthine schwannoma. The actual pathologic substrate for Meniere's disease is dilatation of the endolymphatic spaces owing to a failure of the endolymphatic sac to resorb endolymph. It therefore makes sense that an inflammatory cause (possibly due to a viral infection) of the poor function of the sac might be associated with gadolinium enhancement. Rupture of the cochlear membranes such that perilymph and endolymph mix might cause the sensorineural hearing loss.

Notes

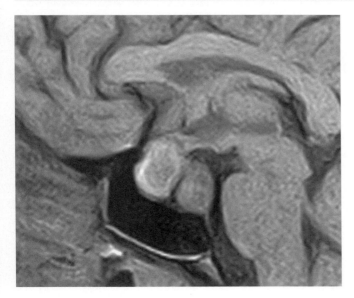

1. Is this patient's history of diabetes insipidus and panhypopituitarism consistent with an anterior pituitary adenoma?

2. What does the history of diabetes insipidus and panhypopituitarism suggest?

3. What is the most common posterior pituitary tumor?

4. Absence of the pituitary bright spot may be seen in what conditions?

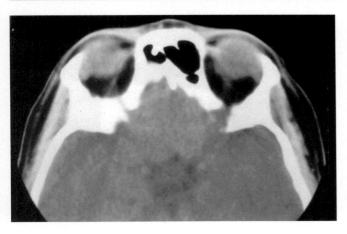 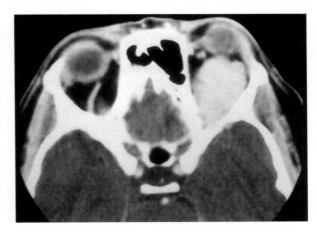

1. What happened between the figure on the left and the figure on the right?

2. What other lesions may expand in a similar fashion?

3. Is the superior ophthalmic vein always involved with varices of the orbit?

4. How would this lesion respond if the patient were maneuvered from a supine flat axial position to a "hanging head" supine hyperextended position?

Pituitary Adenoma and Granular Cell Tumor of the Neurohypophysis

1. No, that would be very unusual.

2. That the lesion affects or is derived from the posterior pituitary or pituitary stalk or that they are affected.

3. Myoblastoma (granular cell tumor, choristoma).

4. Myoblastoma, hemosiderosis, partial volume averaging, ectopic location, diabetes insipidus, histiocytosis X.

Reference

Ji CH, Teng MM, Chang T: Granular cell tumour of the neurohypophysis, *Neuroradiology* 37:451-452, 1995.

Reference

Neuroradiology: THE REQUISITES, pp 313-315, 318.

Comment

The posterior pituitary tumors go by lots of names, including granular cell tumors, granular cell myoblastomas, pituicytomas (owing to their presumed origin from the glial cells of the neurohypophysis), and choristomas. They are benign tumors situated in a tenuous position because they may affect the optic nerves and chiasm. They are relatively hypervascular masses and therefore enhance avidly—in fact, they may bleed uncontrollably at surgery, making a transsphenoidal approach to the tumor somewhat precarious. When a patient has central diabetes insipidus, the high intensity of the posterior pituitary bright spot disappears—this is a pretty good marker of hormonal activity.

The most common tumor in the posterior aspect of the sella is a pituitary adenoma. Give yourself credit if you said that this is just an unusual pituitary adenoma. However, once offered the history in Question 1, you should shift gears to question a posterior neurohypophyseal mass. Gangliogliomas, gangliocytomas, germ cell tumors, craniopharyngiomas, and metastases have also been reported to affect the neurohypophysis.

Notes

Orbital Venous Varix

1. The patient performed a Valsalva maneuver.

2. Dural vascular malformations, hemangiomas, cephaloceles, and neurofibromatosis I (sphenoid wing dysplasia with transmitted CSF changes).

3. No, not always, but it is common.

4. It would expand.

Reference

Yeatts RP, Driver PJ: Orbital varix, *Arch Ophthalmol* 111:702-703, 1993.

Cross-Reference

Neuroradiology: THE REQUISITES, p 294.

Comment

Orbital varices are a cause of unilateral intermittent proptosis. They usually are positional and respond to changes in venous return that can be manipulated by patient positioning in the scanner or via Valsalva or Müller maneuvers. The lesion may spontaneously bleed into the orbit. Phleboliths have been reported.

Some have advocated sonographic evaluation of these lesions. The direction and rate of flow through the dilated vein may be determined in this fashion, so that the differentiation of varices from AVFs or malformations can be made.

The differential diagnosis is an orbital hemangioma. Blue rubber bleb nevus syndrome, a rare cutaneovisceral hemangiomatosis, is associated with vascular lesions of the orbit, particularly hemangiomas.

Notes

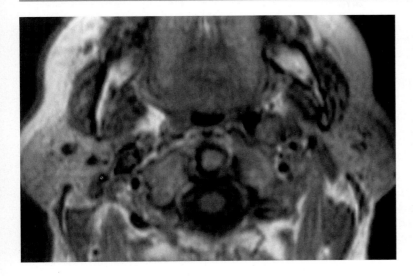
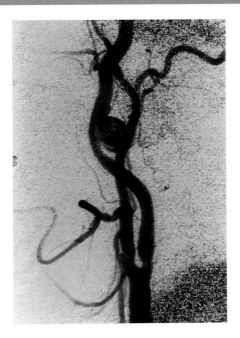

1. In what space is this lesion?

2. What percent of paragangliomas metastasize?

3. The mixed signal intensity of this lesion, with a laminated appearance, should raise the possibility of what diagnosis?

4. When do aneurysms in this location occur?

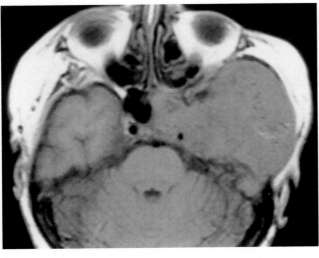
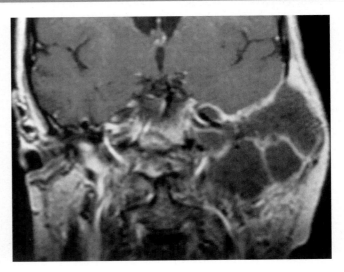

1. What are the two types of acquired cholesteatomas, and how do they differ?

2. Can erosion of the ossicles occur in acute otitis media?

3. Which cholesteatoma (pars tensa or pars flaccida) is more likely to extend into the aditus ad antrum and mastoid air cells?

4. What is the most common place for a congenital cholesteatoma of the temporal bone?

Pseudoaneurysm of the Carotid Artery

1. The carotid space (poststyloid parapharyngeal space).

2. Less than 5%.

3. An aneurysm of the internal carotid artery cervical portion. Partial thrombosis is likely.

4. Posttraumatically, postoperatively, iatrogenically from punctures in the neck, and after dissection. They can also occur in patients who have a collagen deficiency disorder or fibromuscular dysplasia.

Reference

Weissman JL, Johnson JT, Snyderman CH, Steed DL: Thrombosed aneurysm of the cervical carotid artery: avoiding a retrospective diagnosis, *Radiology* 190:869-871, 1994.

Cross-Reference

Neuroradiology: THE REQUISITES, pp 431-432.

Comment

This is an unusual lesion, and the point to be made is that a vagal (or sympathetic plexus) schwannoma or a glomus tumor is a much more likely diagnosis in a patient who has a carotid sheath mass. A glomus tumor enhances uniformly and (hopefully) has flow voids on MRI. A schwannoma may have cystic, nonenhancing areas and may be more heterogeneous than a glomus tumor—differentiating this from an aneurysm may require an MRA or some flow-sensitive pulse sequence. Most of the cervical aneurysms or pseudoaneurysms I have seen in this location have not been completely thrombosed, so some flow should be seen. Blood products and peripheral calcification are unusual in a schwannoma but possible in an aneurysm. Vagal schwannomas displace the carotid and jugular vessels anteriorly and splay them apart. Pseudoaneurysms may occur as a complication of cervical adenitis, peritonsillar abscesses, or deep space neck infections.

Stents are being used more and more frequently to treat pseudoaneurysms in the neck to exclude the lesions from the circulation. In dissected vessels this is a particularly good means for ensuring that the native vessel stays open but the aneurysm is closed. The aneurysm is not so much at risk to rupture as it is as a source of emboli to the intracranial circulation. The alternative, in a patient who has an intact circle of Willis and who passes a balloon occlusion test, is to permanently occlude the damaged vessel. Pseudoaneurysms hardly ever heal themselves.

Notes

Acquired Cholesteatoma

1. The pars flaccida cholesteatoma occurs as a result of perforation through the pars flaccida of the tympanic membrane with accumulation of keratin debris and squamous epithelium in Prussak's space in the epitympanic space, eroding the scutum and malleus. The pars tensa cholesteatoma is less common and affects the inferior portion of the tympanic membrane, leading to involvement of the sinus tympani and distal incus.

2. Yes.

3. The pars flaccida cholesteatoma. Pars tensa cholesteatomas are associated with ossicular erosion in 90% of cases; pars flaccida cholesteatomas in 75%.

4. In the middle ear–mastoid area.

Reference

Liu DP, Bergeron RT: Contemporary radiologic imaging in the evaluation of middle ear–attic–antral complex cholesteatomas, *Otolaryngol Clin North Am* 22:897-910, 1989.

Cross-Reference

Neuroradiology: THE REQUISITES, p 343.

Comment

This patient with a 15-year history of a draining left ear was known to have a cholesteatoma but refused surgical treatment. Eventually the cholesteatoma grew through her temporal bone into her sphenoid sinus, and white cheesy stuff started to drain into her nasopharynx. Ultimately she underwent a huge resection of the cholesteatoma, leaving material in her cavernous sinus and around her fifth cranial nerve. Unfortunately, the pathologists found a microscopic focus of squamous cell carcinoma in the lesion (give yourself partial microscopic credit if you called this case cancer—I cannot argue with you). Note the peripheral enhancement of the lesion, as well as the dural reaction on the coronal scan (figure on right).

Cholesteatomas tend to collect in Prussak's space medial to the scutum and lateral to the neck of the malleus. Therefore the pars flaccida cholesteatoma deviates the ossicles medially. In the absence of erosions, cholesteatomas can look exactly like chronic granulation tissue, chronic otitis media, and middle ear effusions. Look for widening, erosions, and/or displacements of the ossicles, facial nerve, mastoid air cells, Prussak's space, aditus ad antrum, and tegmen tympani. With pars tensa cholesteatomas the ossicles may be displaced laterally, and the epicenter of the lesion may be at the sinus tympani. External auditory canal acquired cholesteatomas usually occur in association with external auditory canal stenosis or atresia.

Notes

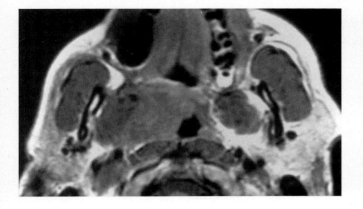
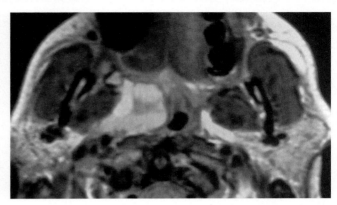
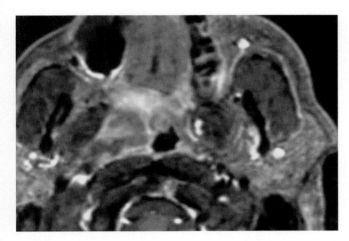

1. What does the differential diagnosis of a prestyloid parapharyngeal space mass include?

2. Why is the term "head and neck synovial sarcoma" considered a misnomer?

3. What are the hallmarks of synovial sarcomas, as opposed to other soft tissue tumors?

4. In the head and neck, what is the most common site of synovial sarcomas?

Parapharyngeal Space Mass—Synovial Sarcoma

1. Minor salivary gland tumor (pleomorphic adenoma, adenoid cystic carcinoma), neurogenic tumor, hemangioma, node, and branchial cleft cyst.

2. The lesion does not arise from joints but has a histologic appearance that simulates synovial cells.

3. Cyst formation, hemorrhage, calcification, loculation, and well-defined borders.

4. The hypopharynx.

Reference

Hirsch RJ, Yousem DM, Loevner LA, Montone KT, Chalian AA, Hayden RE: Synovial sarcomas of the head and neck: MR findings, *AJR Am J Roentgenol* 169:1185-1188, 1997.

Cross-Reference

Neuroradiology: THE REQUISITES, pp 429-431.

Comment

Synovial sarcomas are aggressive, malignant, soft tissue tumors that occur primarily in young adults. They represent 8% to 10% of all soft tissue malignancies, with 85% occurring in the extremities. In the head and neck these lesions favor the hypopharynx and parapharyngeal or masticator space, although reports of lesions in the sinonasal cavity abound. A synovial sarcoma on T1W imaging is most frequently isointense to gray matter and has similar intensity to fat/glandular tissue on T2W scanning. When one encounters these intensity characteristics in a well-defined yet heterogeneous nonmucosal lesion that also contains septations, hemorrhage, cyst formation, calcification, and/or multilocularity, one should consider the diagnosis of synovial sarcoma.

The tumors arise from the mesenchyme and are composed of fibrous connective tissue and synovia-like cells; the former is represented by a spindle cell fibrosarcoma-like component, and the latter are represented by a pseudoepithelial component. However, monophasic varieties of synovial sarcomas (one cell type) have also been described using the term spindle cell sarcomas or epithelioid sarcomas. Spindle cell tumors are difficult to characterize at cytology—histologic specimens for special stains (the mantra of the pathologist) are required.

Notes

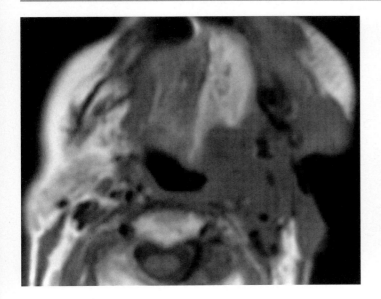
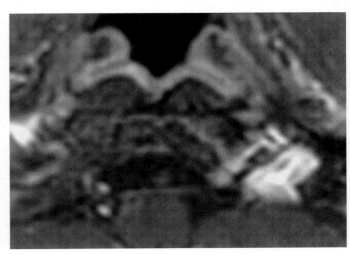
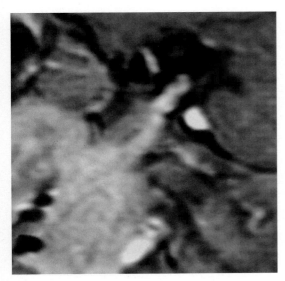

1. The figures provided demonstrate invasion of which neural structures?

2. What are the secondary findings associated with the perineural extension of tumor?

3. Which histologic subtype of malignancy has the greatest propensity for perineural spread of tumor?

4. Perineural extension of tumor is seen in the head and neck most frequently with what tumor?

Adenoid Cystic Carcinoma with Perineural Extension

1. The facial nerve's intramastoid portion and the hypoglossal nerve in the hypoglossal canal.

2. There is tongue atrophy and atrophy of the facial musculature.

3. Adenoid cystic carcinoma (50% to 60%).

4. Squamous cell carcinoma (because it occurs so much more frequently than adenoid cystic carcinoma).

Reference

Sigal R, Monnet O, de Baere T, Micheau C, Shapeero LG, Julieron M, Bosq J, Vanel D, Piekarski J-D, Luboinski B, Masselot J: Adenoid cystic carcinoma of the head and neck: evaluation with MR imaging and clinical-pathologic correlation in 27 patients, *Radiology* 184:95-101, 1992.

Cross-Reference

Neuroradiology: THE REQUISITES, pp 384, 422.

Comment

Adenoid cystic carcinomas account for 5-15% of all salivary gland tumors, 25-31% of malignant minor salivary gland lesions, and 15% of submandibular gland tumors. Adenoid cystic carcinomas with low signal intensity on T2W scans tend to be more cellular than those that have high intensity on T2W scans. The more highly cellular adenoid cystic carcinomas have a worse prognosis than those with less cellularity, so MRI to an extent can predict prognosis. In Sigal et al series, 6 cases had predominantly high T_2W intensity, 9 had intermediate intensity, and 12 had low intensity. Half were heterogenous. In the salivary glands T2W scans are not that reliable in predicting benignity versus malignancy. Sarcomas, low grade mucoepidermoid carcinomas, some adenoid cystic carcinomas, some adenocarcinomas, and some lymphomas are bright on T2W scans. On the other hand, it is the very rare squamous cell carcinoma of the head and neck that is bright on T2W scanning.

Notes

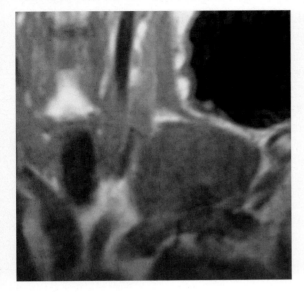 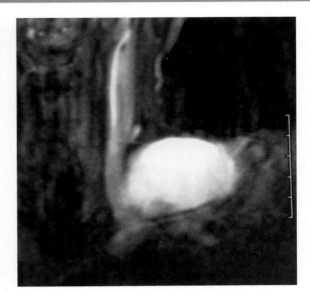

1. Where is this lesion located?

2. Is the lesion cystic or solid?

3. What does the differential diagnosis of a cystic lesion in this location include?

4. What features of branchial cleft cysts make it less likely that this lesion represents such a cyst?

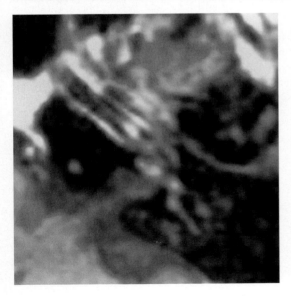 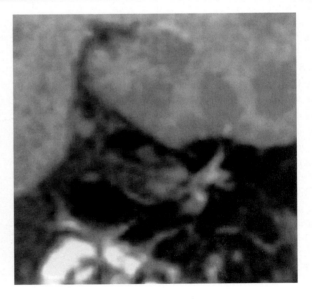

1. What structures are enhancing on this scan?

2. What does the differential diagnosis of labyrinthine enhancement include?

3. What is the classic diagnosis with bilateral internal auditory canal enhancing lesions?

4. Which portion of the cochlea is associated with high frequency hearing loss, and which is associated with low frequency hearing loss?

CASE 162

Cyst in the Lower Neck: Thoracic Duct Lymphocele (Jugular Lymphatic Sac)

1. At the junction between the left jugular vein and the left subclavian vein in the posterolateral compartment of the neck.

2. Cystic (verified by aspiration).

3. Lymphangioma (cystic hygroma), dermoid cyst, lymphocele, necrotic/cystic lymph node, and branchial cleft cyst.

4. Branchial cleft cysts are usually anterior to the sternocleidomastoid muscle and are centered at the level of the angle of the mandible and/or carotid bifurcation.

Reference

Zadvinskis DP, Benson MT, Kerr HH, Mancuso AA, Cacciarelli AA, Madrazo BL, Mafee MF, Dalen K: Congenital malformations of the cervicothoracic lymphatic system: embryology and pathogenesis, *Radiographics* 12:1175-1189, 1992.

Cross-Reference

Neuroradiology: THE REQUISITES, pp 403-405, 431.

Comment

Jugular lymph sac malformations are rare entities that occur as a result of jugular lymphatic obstruction (usually congenital or postoperative). The congenital ones occur during the eighth to ninth week of gestational age, the time when the primitive left juguloaxillary sac connects to the internal jugular vein. The juguloaxillary sac ultimately connects with the thoracic duct at 9 to 10 weeks of gestational age. Lymphangiomas may arise from this area with or without a mature lymphatic system—the theories are that lymphangiomas form when (1) lymphatic ducts do not make it to the venous system, (2) there is sequestered lymphatic tissue, and (3) abnormal budding of lymph vessels occurs, forming cysts that maintain growth potential.

The key to the suggestion of this diagnosis is the location of the lesion where the thoracic duct enters the jugular vein. I have seen two of these, and both have had slightly high signal intensity on T1W scans suggesting hyperproteinaceous contents. This one was aspirated and contained lymph. Thoracic duct or lymphatic vessel injury is not that unusual in head and neck surgery. Having a big cyst like this is peculiar, however.

Notes

CASE 163

Autoimmune Labyrinthitis

1. The cochlea, vestibule, and semicircular canals.

2. Viral labyrinthitis, syphilitic labyrinthitis, Lyme disease, schwannomas, perilymphatic fistulas, trauma, and autoimmune labyrinthitis.

3. Neurofibromatosis type 2 (central NF).

4. High frequency hearing loss is usually seen with basilar turn cochlear enhancement, whereas low frequency hearing loss is usually seen with apical turn cochlear enhancement.

Reference

Mark AS, Fitzgerald D: Segmental enhancement of the cochlea on contrast-enhanced MR: correlation with the frequency of hearing loss and possible sign of perilymphatic fistula and autoimmune labyrinthitis, *AJNR Am J Neuroradiol* 14:991-996, 1993.

Cross-Reference

Neuroradiology: THE REQUISITES, pp 352-353.

Comment

Complete hearing loss may also be seen with basilar turn enhancement. After ruling out a schwannoma because of absence of enlargement of the cochlea and resolution of the enhancement with steroid therapy, one is left with autoimmune labyrinthitis, viral labyrinthitis, and perilymphatic fistulas as possible causes of selective cochlear turn enhancement. Lymphocytic reaction to inner ear antigen may lead to attacks on the scala tympani of the cochlea and round window membrane in autoimmune labyrinthitis. The entity is usually responsive to steroid therapy. Bacterial causes of labyrinthitis are usually the result of spread from the middle ear or meningitis.

Notes

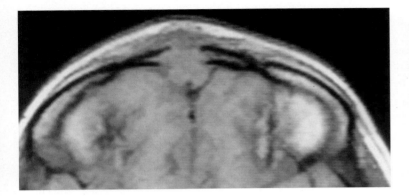
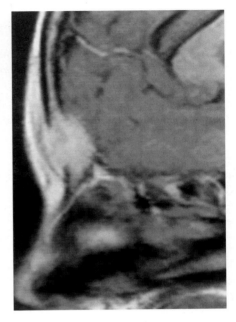

1. In a 12-year-old boy, what diagnoses should be entertained for this intranasal/extranasal mass?

2. How can the diagnoses from Question 1 be distinguished based on enhancement characteristics?

3. What are the most common sites of Langerhans cell histiocytosis (eosinophilic granuloma) in the skull base?

4. What are the classic features of Langerhans cell histiocytosis in the calvaria?

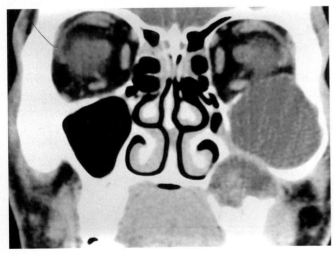
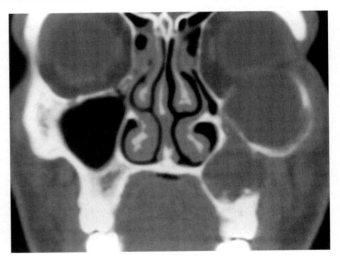

1. What are the two most common cysts of odontogenic origin?

2. What are the imaging characteristics of odontogenic keratocysts?

3. Are odontogenic keratocysts associated with unerupted teeth?

4. Describe the syndrome associated with odontogenic keratocysts.

Eosinophilic Granuloma of the Nasofrontal Region

1. Meningoencephaloceles, nasal gliomas, hemangiomas, dermoid sinus tracts, sarcomas, eosinophilic granuloma, and rhabdomyosarcoma.

2. Meningoencephaloceles, nasal gliomas, and dermoid sinus tracts should not enhance, whereas the other inflammatory and neoplastic lesions usually do enhance.

3. The temporal bones, the mandible, and the bony calvaria.

4. Punched-out well-defined lesions in the skull with beveled edges and no associated sclerosis.

Reference

Siegelman SS: Taking the X out of Histiocytosis X, *Radiology* 204:322-324, 1997.

Cross-Reference

Neuroradiology: THE REQUISITES, p 354.

Comment

Langerhans cells are created in the bone marrow and are derived from CD34+ stem cells. They are commonly found in the skin, lungs, thymus, and lymph nodes, where they help to process antigens for the T lymphocytes. The pathology of Langerhans cell histiocytosis is due to a proliferation and deregulation of these cells in the bone, skin, nodes, and lung most commonly. Inflammatory eosinophils and monocytes may also be present, and after a while a fibrotic reaction is the end result of the Langerhans cell infiltrate.

Eosinophilic granuloma, Letterer-Siwe disease, and Hand-Schüller-Christian disease comprise the spectrum of illnesses encapsulated by Langerhans cell histiocytosis. The hypothalamus and/or neurohypophysis is the most common site of intracranial involvement. Meningeal involvement may also be present, but calvarial disease is the most common manifestation in the head and neck. Scalp rashes, mandibular lesions, adenopathy, and gingival ulcers may also be present with this disorder of childhood. Treatment options include steroids, low-dose radiation, and surgery as needed.

Radiologists are used to dealing with Langerhans cell histiocytosis (histiocytosis X) in discussing lesions of the pituitary stalk that cause diabetes insipidus. Langerhans cell histiocytosis is a cause of loss of the pituitary bright spot (which correlates with symptoms of diabetes insipidus). Strong enhancement is common. After the hypothalamus and pituitary gland, the cerebellum is the most common intraaxial site of Langerhans cell histiocytosis. The lesion is relatively radiosensitive.

Notes

Keratocyst

1. Dentigerous (follicular) and periapical (radicular) cysts.

2. They are usually multilocular cysts that occur most commonly in the mandible (67%) and grow aggressively but that have smooth, scalloped borders with thin sclerotic margins. They grow in an anteroposterior direction and often preserve cortical margins.

3. Less commonly than dentigerous cysts.

4. Basal cell nevus syndrome (Gorlin's syndrome)—an autosomal dominant syndrome that is associated with multiple odontogenic keratocysts, marked calcification of the falx and dura of the brain, multiple basal cell carcinomas of the skin, pitting of the skin of the palm, and bifid ribs.

Reference

Minami M, Kaneda T, Ozawa K, Yamamoto H, Itai Y, Ozawa M, Yoshikawa K, Sasaki Y: Cystic lesions of the maxillomandibular region: MR imaging distinction of odontogenic keratocysts and ameloblastomas from other cysts, *AJR Am J Roentgenol* 166:943-949, 1996.

Cross-Reference

Neuroradiology: THE REQUISITES, pp 389-390.

Comment

Odontogenic keratocysts account for about one tenth of all cystic lesions of the jaw and are far outnumbered by dentigerous (follicular) and radicular (periapical) cysts. They favor the third molar region, similar to dentigerous cysts. They favor the mandible over the maxilla by a 4:1 margin. Included in the differential diagnosis are ameloblastoma, aneurysmal bone cyst, myxoma, giant cell tumor, cherubism, and atypical dentigerous cyst. At the mandibular molar region the differential diagnosis is usually between odontogenic keratocyst and ameloblastoma—if the tooth root is resorbed and the cortex is expanded, favor an ameloblastoma; if the walls are thin and the lesion does not enhance much, favor an odontogenic keratocyst. If the lesion grows in an anteroposterior direction without expanding the cortex, favor an odontogenic keratocyst. The fluid in an odontogenic keratocyst is said to be of higher intensity on T1W MRI and lower intensity on T2W MRI than the fluid in an ameloblastoma. Recurrence rates for odontogenic keratocysts are high (up to 60%). When there are multiple odontogenic keratocysts, basal cell nevus syndrome is present in 50% of cases.

Notes

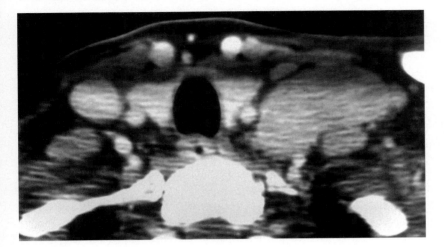

1. What is the differential diagnosis of this low cervical lesion?

2. Marked contrast-enhancing lymph nodes occur in what disease processes?

3. What are the typical locations of Castleman's disease?

4. What is angiofollicular lymph node hyperplasia?

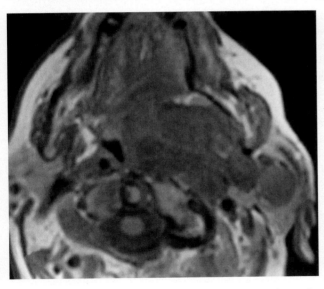 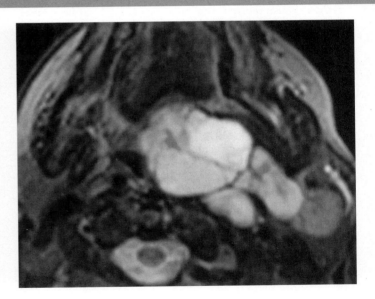

1. What is the recurrence rate of a pleomorphic adenoma?

2. If the pleomorphic adenoma is not resected, what is the expected rate of malignant degeneration?

3. What are the issues related to seeding of pleomorphic adenomas?

4. What is the most common location of pleomorphic adenomas of the minor salivary gland?

CASE 166

Castleman's Disease

1. Schwannoma, hemangioma, neurofibroma, lymphoma, or other lymph node disease.

2. Metastatic thyroid carcinoma, Castleman's disease, metastatic Kaposi's carcinoma, and some forms of lymphoma.

3. The abdomen (20%) is second to the mediastinum (70%). The neck is a relatively uncommon location (<10%).

4. Another name for Castleman's disease (also giant lymph node hyperplasia).

Reference

Glazer M, Rao VM, Reiter D, McCue P: Isolated Castleman disease of the neck: MR findings, *AJNR Am J Neuroradiol* 16:669-671, 1995.

Cross-Reference

Neuroradiology: THE REQUISITES, p 405.

Comment

Most cases (76% to 91%) of localized Castleman's disease are of the hyaline vascular type, which tends to have a favorable prognosis and course. Patients are in their 30s at the time of onset. The mediastinum and neck are the preferred sites of the hyaline vascular subtype. Alternatively, one may have the plasma cell variant, which is associated with "B" symptoms of lymphoma—fever, anemia, weight loss, and so on. Elevated IgGs to Epstein-Barr virus antigens are found. The patients are younger than those with the hyaline vascular type, and the mesenteric and retroperitoneal nodes are preferentially affected. There often is a central low density, low intensity area within the lymph nodes that may represent fibrosis and may point to the correct diagnosis. Surgery is the preferred treatment, but radiation and steroid therapy are also curative. The generalized forms of Castleman's disease (nonneuropathic and neuropathic varieties) have a far worse prognosis with a greater risk of succumbing to infections or dedifferentiation into a lymphoma or Kaposi's sarcoma. The patients affected with the multicentric varieties of the disease are older and more commonly men. Note that this mass is anterior to the scalene musculature and therefore unassociated with the brachial plexus. This might suggest a diagnosis other than a schwannoma, which was the primary differential in this case.

Notes

CASE 167

Seeding of a Parotid Pleomorphic Adenoma

1. Approximately 15% to 20%.

2. Twenty percent to 25%.

3. Because cutting through the lesion carries the risk of creating seeds of the tumor, it is important to perform a wide local parotidectomy and not to rupture the capsule of the tumor during resection. Additionally, small-gauge needles (20 gauge or smaller) are recommended for aspirations of these tumors.

4. The palate.

Reference

Ikeda K, Katoh T, Ha-Kawa SK, Iwai H, Yamashita T, Tanaka Y: The usefulness of MR in establishing the diagnosis of parotid pleomorphic adenoma, *AJNR Am J Neuroradiol* 17:555-559, 1996.

Cross-Reference

Neuroradiology: THE REQUISITES, pp 385-386, 419-420, 424.

Comment

Pleomorphic adenomas, by and large, are well-defined, encapsulated masses that abound in all sites of salivary gland tissue. They often have lobulated margins and almost always are bright on T2W scans. A complete capsule is seen in 82% of parotid pleomorphic adenomas and 15% of parotid malignancies. Forty-two percent of malignant tumors have well-defined margins. Thirty-four percent of malignant parotid masses have high signal intensity on T2W scans. If a lesion has a well-defined, complete capsule and a lobulated contour, the positive predictive value for a pleomorphic adenoma or benign parotid mass is close to 100%. Recurrence of pleomorphic adenoma of the parotid usually occurs in the operative bed. Extensive seeding in the parotid bed is not that uncommon, but seeding in the neck is reportable. Because of the high rate of malignant transformation, combined radical surgery and radiotherapy are recommended for many patients who have recurrences. This case would be hard to cure with surgery alone.

The presence of fat or calcification in a parotid mass favors the diagnosis of pleomorphic adenoma, though such pleomorphic adenomas are found infrequently in comparison with other pleomorphic adenomas.

Notes

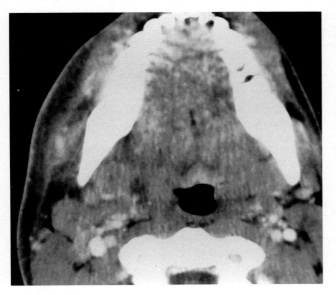 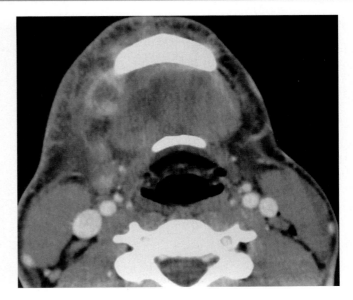

1. What is the classic organism associated with this condition?

2. What is the prognosis?

3. Are areas of gas collection unusual in the lesion?

4. Are areas of multiloculation unusual in the entity?

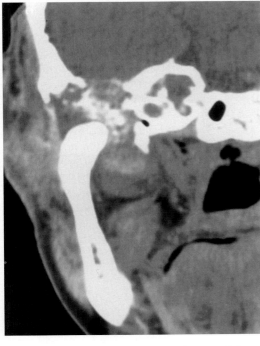 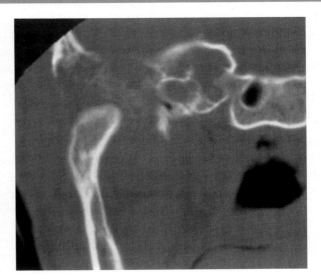

1. Are lesions of the mandibular condyle more commonly classified as odontogenic lesions or true bone lesions?

2. What are the common malignancies of the mandibular condyle?

3. What are the benign aggressive lesions of the temporomandibular joint?

4. A lytic lesion of the condylar head that does not affect the distal end of the bone can be seen with what lesions?

Necrotizing Fasciitis

1. Group A ß-hemolytic *Streptococcus* more so than *Staphylococcus,* but mixed aerobic and anaerobic infections are also not uncommon.

2. This is a rapidly fatal disease. It must be diagnosed early.

3. No.

4. No.

Reference

Becker M, Zbaren P, Hermans R, Becker CD, Marchal F, Kurt A-M, Marre S, Rufenacht DA, Terrier F: Necrotizing fasciitis of the head and neck: role of CT in diagnosis and management, *Radiology* 202:471-476, 1997.

Cross-Reference

Neuroradiology: THE REQUISITES, pp 424-427.

Comment

This disease has seen an explosion in the late 1980s and 1990s and is a scary entity. The mortality is over 70%, and the patients may undergo a horrifying sloughing of skin and subcutaneous tissue that leaves huge scars. Initially the etiology and organism were not clearly identified because the dermal entry site is usually a pretty minor infection. Now with early surgical intervention (antibiotics are insufficient for treatment), the cure rates are much better. The CT findings in this disease include cellulitic infiltration of the skin and subcutaneous tissues, cervical fascial thickening and enhancement, muscular thickening and enhancement, multicompartmental fluid collections, gas collections (due to anaerobic bacteria populations) and associated mediastinitis, and pleural empyemas. Histopathologically, the entity induces a vasculitis and small vessel thromboses. An odontogenic or pharyngeal cause may be present if no skin entry portal is present. The main distinction between a cellulitis and/or abscess and necrotizing fasciitis is the asymmetric thickening and enhancement of the muscles and investing cervical fascia (deep and superficial) around the various spaces of the neck in necrotizing fasciitis.

Notes

Chondroblastoma of the Temporal Bone, Temporomandibular Joint

1. Usually true bone lesions.

2. Metastases, myeloma, osteosarcoma, Ewing's sarcoma, and chondrosarcoma.

3. Rheumatoid arthritis, pigmented villonodular synovitis, synovial chondromatosis, synovioma, brown tumor, and giant cell reparative granuloma.

4. Unicameral bone cyst, aneurysmal bone cyst, osteoblastoma, and chondroblastoma.

Reference

Flowers CH, Rodriguez J, Naseem M, Reyes MM, Verano AS: MR of benign chondroblastoma of the temporal bone, *AJNR Am J Neuroradiol* 16:414-416, 1995.

Cross-Reference

Neuroradiology: THE REQUISITES, pp 424-427.

Comment

This case was thought to arise in the temporal bone and secondarily affect the temporomandibular joint. The temporal bone is an unusual site for a chondroblastoma. Chondroblastomas usually occur in the epiphyses of long bones. Nonetheless, in the skull the temporal bone is the most common location. Males are affected more commonly than females—those under 20 years of age are usually affected by a lesion in the humerus and tibia, but middle-aged adults are at risk for a lesion occurring in the skull. Calcification is seen in 30% to 50% of cases. Inhomogeneous signal intensity is the norm on MRI pulse sequences, especially T2W scans. The presence of calcification and cartilage histologically probably accounts for the heterogeneity of density and intensity. Treatment is surgical.

Give yourself credit if you thought the diagnosis was a chondrosarcoma (my preoperative diagnosis, to be honest). The risk factors for developing a head and neck sarcoma include prior irradiation, association with retinoblastoma (oncogene), Paget's disease, and fibrous dysplasia. Histopathologically, it is often difficult to distinguish benign from malignant chondroid lesions of the head and neck. Metastases from chondrosarcoma are rare, but local recurrence is common. The nasal septum is a common site of chondrosarcomas—much more so than the temporomandibular joint and the cricoid cartilage (even though the latter is a roentgen classic!).

Notes

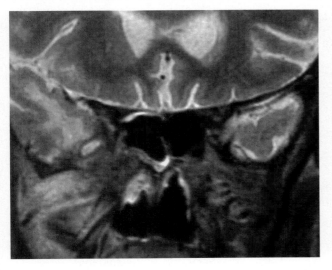
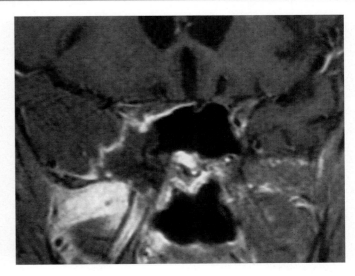

1. What are the typical imaging features of fungal sinus infections?

2. What is the most common fungus found in the paranasal sinuses?

3. Describe the different forms of aspergillosis that may affect the sinonasal cavity.

4. What is the typical finding on potassium hydroxide staining for *Aspergillus?*

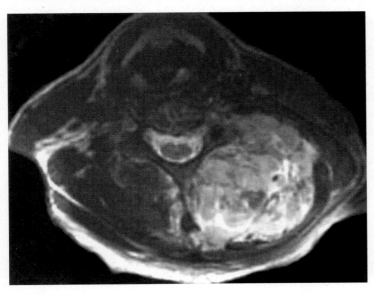
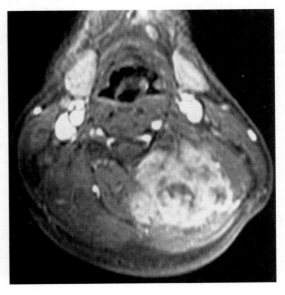

1. What diagnoses could be considered with this large mass in the posterior musculature?

2. What argues against this being an inflammatory mass?

3. What are the most common nonneurogenic soft tissue tumors in the pediatric and adult age groups to affect the head and neck?

4. What type of lymphoma infiltrates soft tissue?

Aspergillosis of the Skull Base

1. They may be hypointense, isointense, or hyperintense on T1W scans; dark on T2W scans; and hyperdense on CT.

2. Aspergillus

3. One can have (1) an acute/fulminant (invasive) form, (2) a chronic/indolent (invasive) form, (3) a fungus ball, and (4) an allergic fungal sinusitis.

4. Less than 45-degree branching septate hyphae.

Reference

McLean FM, Ginsberg LE, Stanton CA: Perineural spread of rhinocerebral mucormycosis, *AJNR Am J Neuroradiol* 17: 114-116, 1996.

Cross-Reference

Neuroradiology: THE REQUISITES, pp 192-193.

Comment

Fungal sinusitis is separated into invasive and noninvasive forms. The invasive forms include an acute fulminant variety, usually seen in immunosuppressed individuals (such as this patient with AIDS), and a chronic indolent form. Of the noninvasive variety, fungus balls and allergic fungal sinusitis are the main subtypes. The acute fulminant type may have hematogenous spread via the cavernous sinus, with aspergillosis—or more commonly mucormycosis—of the sinonasal cavity. This is a devastating illness that has orbital and intracranial ramifications if not treated urgently—a cause for an emergency imaging study. I have also seen pseudoaneurysms develop due to fungal sinusitis. Finally, one can have perineural spread of the fungal infection in addition to angiotropic growth.

Allergic fungal sinusitis is characterized by the presence of "allergic mucin," with scattered fungal organisms, eosinophilia, and no invasion of mucosa or bone. That said, there have been scattered reports of skull base erosion with allergic fungal sinusitis. The organisms involved are fungi of the Dematiaceae family (*Bipolaris, Curvularia* genera). On imaging one sees high density (with or without calcifications) on CT and low intensity on T2W corresponding to thick inspissated allergic mucin.

Notes

Lymphoma of the Soft Tissues

1. Sarcomas, neurofibromas, fibromatoses, lymphoma, hemangiopericytoma, and MFH.

2. The absence of edema and stranding in the subcutaneous tissues.

3. Rhabdomyosarcomas in children and fibrous lesions (MFH, fibrosarcomas, desmoids, fibromas, nodular fasciitis, and fibrous histiocytoma) in adults.

4. Non-Hodgkin's lymphoma.

Reference

Lee VS, Martinez S, Coleman RE: Primary muscle lymphoma, *Radiology* 203:237-244, 1997.

Cross-Reference

Neuroradiology: THE REQUISITES, pp 406-408.

Comment

Lymphoma is the second most common malignancy of the head and neck (after squamous cell carcinoma) and the most common in the 21- to 40-year-old age bracket. Lymphoma in the head and neck may be typed into (1a) unilateral nodal lymphoma, (1b) bilateral nodal lymphoma, (2a) extranodal lymphoma confined to Waldeyer's ring, (2b) extranodal lymphoma outside Waldeyer's ring, (3a) Waldeyer's ring plus nodes, (3b) extralymphatic lymphoma plus nodes, (4a) multifocal extranodal lymphoma without nodes, and (4b) multifocal extranodal lymphoma with nodes. This is a case of 2b disease—outside nodes and Waldeyer's ring. Lymphoma can affect virtually any bone or soft tissue in the head and neck, including the subcutaneous fat, skin, and muscles. Isolated lymphoma to muscle occurs in only 1.4% of all extranodal lymphomas and is usually (as in this case) non-Hodgkin's lymphoma. Metastatic lymphoma to the muscle is, in fact, more common than disease in the muscle alone. Therefore an aggressive search for other sites of lymphoma is warranted. High on the differential diagnosis should be some type of sarcoma and hemangiopericytoma. On MRI all muscular lymphomas should be hyperintense on T2W scans, and the adjacent bone may be free of disease.

Notes

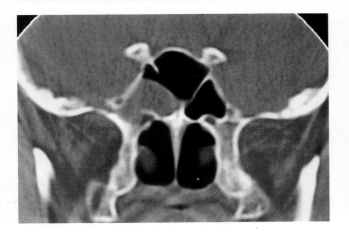

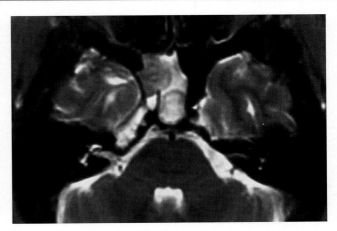

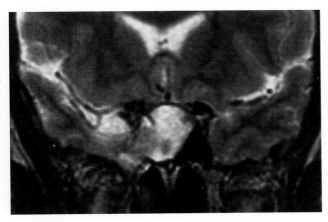

1. What is the difference between a sincipital and a basal encephalocele?

2. What is important to describe when one deals with a meningoencephalocele?

3. What is the most common site of meningo(encephalo)celes?

4. What ethnic group is predisposed to encephaloceles, and where do they occur?

Encephalocele

1. A sincipital encephalocele is visible from the outside, whereas a basal encephalocele is not.

2. What's in the sac. Surgeons like to avoid resecting brain, vessels, and nerves. That stuff is better put back where it belongs.

3. Trick question—the lumbar region (meningo[myelo]-celes). In the head and neck the most common site is probably the occipital region (often as part of the Arnold-Chiari malformation syndrome).

4. Southeast Asians (particularly girls) have a higher rate of sphenoethmoidal encephaloceles. In North America and Australia occipital encephaloceles predominate.

Reference

Czech T, Reinprecht A, Matula C, Svoboda H, Vorkapic P: Cephaloceles: experience with 42 patients, *Acta Neurochirur* 134:125-129, 1995.

Cross-Reference

Neuroradiology: THE REQUISITES, pp 249-250.

Comment

More and more physicians have adopted the term *cephalocele* to generically refer to herniation of intracranial tissues through a cranial defect or the skull base. This seems reasonable, but I will not use the British pronunciation of *k*ephalocele, just as I do not pronounce *c*ephalic as *k*ephalic! Sincipital and basal cephaloceles are nearly equally split in frequency at the skull base. Cleft lip, choanal atresia, hypertelorism, agenesis of the corpus callosum, colobomas, ocular and optic abnormalities, and so on may coexist with the cephalocele. The risk of intracranial coexistent anomalies is much higher with frontal, occipital, and parietal cephaloceles than with basal ones. Posterior encephaloceles have the worst prognosis probably because of the related brain problems and Arnold-Chiari malformation link. CSF leaks are the biggest problem with basal cephaloceles.

Patients with transsphenoidal encephaloceles may present with hormonal dysfunction (growth hormone most commonly), diabetes insipidus, or optic nerve dysfunction, which may progress with time. This patient presented with partial complex seizures, presumably because of traction on the temporal lobe.

Notes

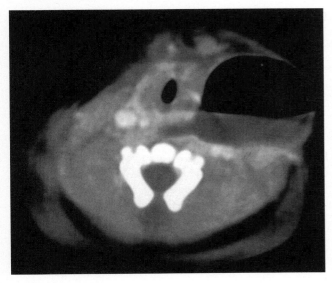

1. What is the most likely cause of this lesion in a newborn?
2. What does the differential diagnosis of an air and fluid–filled lesion in the neck include?
3. Where does each of the branchial cleft fistulas typically drain?
4. What is derived from fourth branchial tissue?

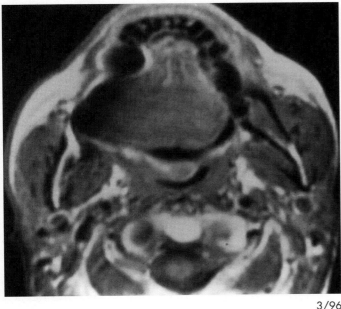
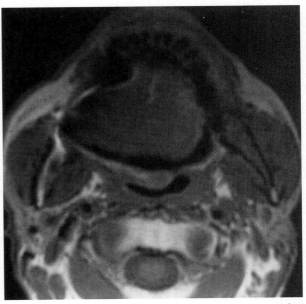

3/96

9/96

1. What is the rate of lymph node metastases from base of tongue carcinoma?
2. How can one distinguish between tumor and osteoradionecrosis?
3. At what radiation dose is the mandible susceptible to osteoradionecrosis?
4. Given the relative lack of change in the marrow and soft tissue surrounding the mandible in these two studies 6 months apart, what is the most likely diagnosis?

Fourth Branchial Cleft Fistula to the Pyriform Sinus

1. A tracheo-esophageal fistula.

2. Pharyngocele, laryngocele, Zenker's diverticulum, duplication cyst, neurenteric cyst, abscess, and branchial cleft cyst with fistula.

3. Type I—to the ear; type II—to the palatine tonsil; type III—to the piriform sinus; and type IV—to the piriform sinus apex.

4. Fourth arch—ultimobranchial bodies, thyroid cartilage, vagus nerve, aortic arch, right subclavian artery, and laryngeal muscles. Fourth cleft—involutes (cervical sinus of His). Fourth pouch—piriform fossa, superior parathyroid tissue.

Reference

Bar-Ziv J, Slasky BS, Sichel JY, Liberman A, Katz R: Branchial pouch sinus tract from the piriform fossa causing acute suppurative thyroiditis, neck abscess, or both: CT appearance and the use of air as a contrast agent, *AJR Am J Roentgenol* 167:1569-1572, 1996.

Cross-Reference

Neuroradiology: THE REQUISITES, pp 336, 393, 416.

Comment

A branchial pouch sinus tract from the piriform sinus may arise from the third or fourth branchial pouch. It is a potential cause of acute suppurative thyroiditis. The tract to the thyroid gland is usually seen in childhood or infancy with painful swelling of the neck, fever, and sore throat. For some reason, this is more often a left-sided process.

If a branchial apparatus anomaly communicates with the skin from the piriform fossa, call it a branchial cleft sinus; if it communicates with the pharynx, call it a branchial pouch sinus; but if it connects from viscus to viscus or viscus to skin, call it a fistula. Persistent mucous drainage from the skin opening is a frequent presenting symptom. The air seen in this case may represent a communication with the pharynx or the presence of an abscess—soft tissue inflammation and infiltration of fat would suggest the latter. Apparently, a third or fourth branchial origin of the sinus tract can be distinguished based on the location of the tract with respect to the superior laryngeal nerve. If the tract passes above the superior laryngeal nerve, it probably came from the third pouch; if below, it probably came from the fourth pouch. Recurrence rates are about 4% to 10%.

The branchial cleft anomalies are often lined by squamous epithelium and contain subepithelial lymphoid tissue. Skin adnexal structures may be seen within the fistula.

Notes

Osteoradionecrosis of the Mandible

1. 70-80%.

2. It is difficult. PET and thallium scanning have been proposed—hot with tumor, not with inflammation.

3. At 6500 rad, 5% of patients develop osteoradionecrosis within 5 years.

4. Radiation fibrosis.

Reference

Chung TS, Yousem DM, Seigerman HS, Hayden RE, Weinstein G: MR of mandibular invasion in patients with oral and oropharyngeal malignant neoplasms, *AJNR Am J Neuroradiol* 15:1949-1955, 1994.

Cross-Reference

Neuroradiology: THE REQUISITES, pp 408-410.

Comment

Diagnosing invasion of the mandible by cancer with MRI is a little tricky. Things like odontogenic infections, radiation fibrosis, osteoradionecrosis, and peritumoral edema can simulate gross replacement of the bone marrow by tumor. MRI suffers more from false positives than false negatives. Subtle cortical invasion that is seen on CT can be detected on MRI using thin-section T1W scans. Give up on CT if the patient has a mouth full of dental amalgam—you may never get a good look at the bone on CT. MRI is better in that setting. Mandibular invasion with oral cavity cancer occurs in 11% to 39% of cases. The site of mandibular invasion is also important because perineural spread is more likely if the mental or inferior alveolar canals are involved. Osteoradionecrosis is treated entirely differently—usually with hyperbaric oxygen and antibiotics. Tumor grows like poison ivy in the setting of hyperbaric oxygen, so this is an important distinction.

Radiation therapy may result in diminished blood supply to the mandible and osteoblastic or osteoclastic activity. Most often CT scans show areas of bony lysis, cortical interruption, and reduced trabeculation, whereas MRI shows the marrow replacement. The entity may be precipitated by such things as dental extractions or infections after radiation therapy. Vascularized flaps may be useful to treat this entity if hyperbaric oxygen fails.

Flaps are usually separated into several categories—site (local, regional, or distant), tissue (cutaneous, fasciocutaneous, myocutaneous, or osteomyocutaneous), and blood supply (random, axial, pedicled, or free). Grafts are free tissue transfers without a vascular supply and necessitate the dermal and subdermal vessels to grow into them to keep them viable.

Notes

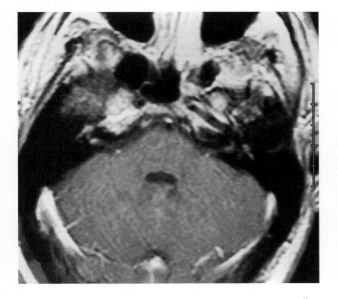
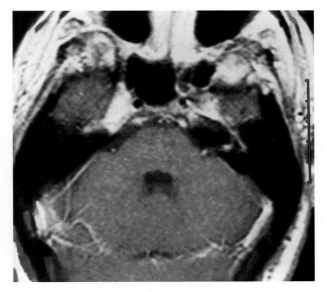
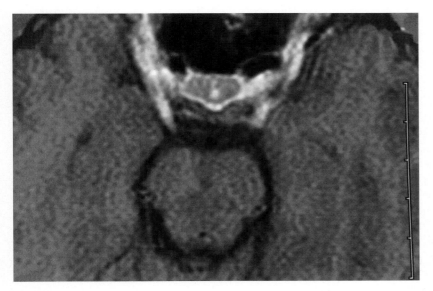

1. What does the differential diagnosis of multiple enhancing enlarged cranial nerves include?

2. What should one consider in the differential diagnosis of peripheral neuronal enlargement?

3. In the presence of pituitary stalk enhancement in this case, what should be considered?

4. True or false: NF type 1 is more commonly associated with peripheral neurogenic tumors than NF type 2.

Multiple Enhancing Cranial Nerves: Dejerine-Sottas Disease

1. Lymphoma, NF, subarachnoid seeding, infections (tuberculosis, *Mycobacterium avium-intracellulare,* Lyme disease, virus), neurodegenerative hypertrophic disorders, and sarcoidosis.

2. Congenital causes (Charcot-Marie-Tooth disease, hereditary motor or sensory neuropathy type III Dejerine-Sottas disease) and neoplasms (neurogenic tumors, lymphoma, perineural spread of tumors, meningioma).

3. Sarcoidosis, mycobacterial infections, lymphoma, subarachnoid seeding, and Wegener's granulomatosis.

4. True.

Reference

Tachi N, Kozuka N, Ohya K, Chiba S, Naganuma M: MRI of peripheral nerves and pathology of sural nerves in hereditary motor and sensory neuropathy type III, *Neuroradiology* 37: 496-499, 1995.

Cross-Reference

Neuroradiology: THE REQUISITES, pp 474, 490.

Comment

Dejerine-Sottas disease is a hereditary polyneuropathy that affects children early in life with hypomyelination of the nerves. It has been associated with mutations of the peripheral myelin protein gene on chromosome 22. Inheritance is usually autosomal recessive. As such, it is usually in the differential diagnosis of Charcot-Marie-Tooth disease because the manifestations are usually in the extremities, not in the CNS. The sural nerve, most commonly affected in the extremities, becomes markedly enlarged and demyelinated and has an "onion bulb" appearance, with rings of demyelination around the central myelinated fibers. Although it is usually a peripheral neuropathy, I have seen two patients with striking enlargement and enhancement of their cranial nerves or intraspinal nerves with Dejerine-Sottas syndrome. Patients usually have weakness and muscle atrophy in the distribution of the affected nerves. Sensation may be affected, leading to Charcot joints.

What you should have noticed in this case are the abnormally enhancing seventh and eighth cranial nerves and mandibular nerves bilaterally in the figures in the upper left and upper right, the large enhancing gasserian ganglion on the right in the figure in the upper right, and the large enhancing third nerve on the right in the figure in the lower left.

Notes

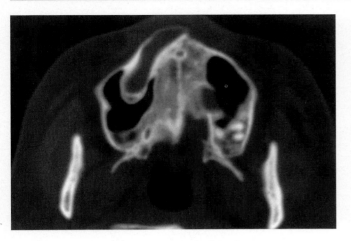 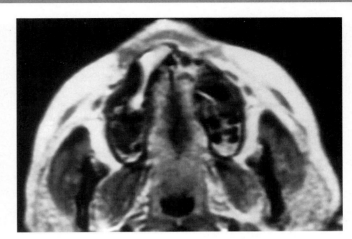

1. Name four congenital maxillofacial cysts.

2. What is the clinical significance of this cyst?

3. The nasopalatine nerve is a branch of what nerve?

4. What structures fail to fuse with median cleft lips, lateral cleft lips, and cleft palates?

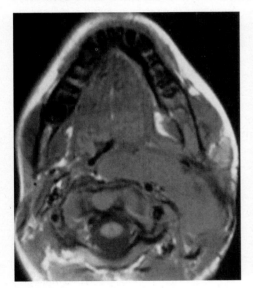 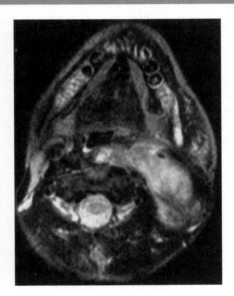

1. What are the typical T2W scan findings with fibromatosis of the neck?

2. Where are the most common locations of fibromatosis in the neck?

3. With what diagnoses is this lesion related?

4. Describe the demographics of this lesion.

Nasoalveolar Cyst

1. Nasopalatine (incisive), nasoalveolar, globulomaxillary, and Stafne cysts.

2. It poses little health risk. Cosmetic issues determine treatment.

3. The second division of the trigeminal nerve (maxillary nerve).

4. Nasomedial processes, nasomedial processes to nasolateral processes, and palatine shelves, respectively.

Reference

Cure JK, Osguthorpe JD, Van Tassel P: MR of nasolabial cysts, *AJNR Am J Neuroradiol* 17:585-588, 1996.

Cross-Reference

Neuroradiology: THE REQUISITES, pp 360-362.

Comment

Nasoalveolar (nasolabial) cysts are extraosseous soft tissue cysts that occur along the lateral nasal alae and represent an inclusion cyst as the nasomedial process and the maxillary processes fuse and the nasolacrimal system is being formed. The cysts occur more commonly in women and are bilateral in 11%. They are seen as protrusions under the upper lip, deep to the mucosa. Their signal intensity is variable on T1W scans and bright on T2W scans. They do not enhance. Crystals and calcium precipitates may occur in the dependent portions of the lesion. The cyst may be lined by pseudostratified columnar epithelium with or without squamous, cuboidal, and goblet cell elements.

Incisive (nasopalatine) canal cysts are intraosseous midline lesions. Globulomaxillary cysts occur between lateral incisor and canine teeth in the maxilla and may extend into the maxillary sinus.

Notes

Fibromatosis of the Neck

1. It is intermediate in intensity but may be dark.

2. Posterior neck and pharynx.

3. Autoimmune fibritides, fibrosarcomas, MFHs, and desmoid tumors.

4. It occurs in young adult females.

Reference

Lewin JS, Lavertu P: Aggressive fibromatosis of the prevertebral and retropharyngeal spaces: MR and CT characteristics, *AJNR Am J Neuroradiol* 16:897-900, 1995.

Cross-Reference

Neuroradiology: THE REQUISITES, p 442.

Comment

Eleven percent of extraabdominal fibromatoses occur in the head and neck. Although benign, fibromatosis of the neck is an aggressive lesion prone to recurrence that is associated with persistent, painless swelling of the soft tissues of the neck. There often is a history of trauma associated with the onset of the lesion. It has also been termed desmoid tumor, musculoaponeurotic fibromatosis, and desmoma, but histologically it represents a soft tissue neoplasm that is poorly defined and is made of collagen and spindle cells.

Nodular fasciitis is the most common head and neck benign mesenchymal tumor in early to late childhood (Kransdorf MJ: Benign soft-tissue tumors in a large referral population: distribution of specific diagnoses by age, sex, and location, *AJR Am J Roentgenol* 164:395-402, 1995), with fibrous histiocytoma closely following (along with hemangiomas). In adults only lipomas predominate over nodular fasciitis and fibrous histiocytoma in the head and neck.

This case crosses the fascial planes of the neck. Medially one sees that the lesion enters the retropharyngeal space in front of the longus colli muscles. It also appears to be anterior to the carotid artery, putting it in the parapharyngeal space. But its lateral extension is in what some call the posterolateral space—which only goes to show, take all of our dogmatic teachings about spaces of the neck with a grain of salt.

Notes

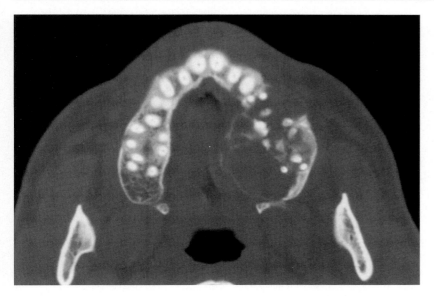

1. With what implant are giant cell reparative granulomas of the mandibular condyle associated?

2. What other processes predispose to giant cell reparative granulomas of the mandible?

3. What other complications are associated with meniscal prostheses?

4. What mandibular lesions are associated with supernumerary teeth?

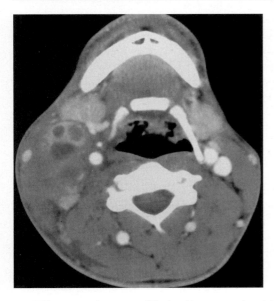

1. What are the most likely diagnoses in this patient?

2. Describe the bacteriology of brucellosis.

3. What is the incidence of head and neck adenopathy in asymptomatic HIV-positive men?

4. What is the incidence of adenopathy in my two children in any month of fall or winter?

Giant Cell Reparative Granuloma of the Maxilla

1. Teflon-Proplast meniscus prostheses.

2. Carious teeth.

3. Granulation tissue, migration, and intracranial extension.

4. Odontomas and Pindborg tumors.

Reference

Uchino A, Kato A, Yonemitsu N, Hirotsu T, Kudo S: Giant cell reparative granuloma of the cranial vault, *AJNR Am J Neuroradiol* 17:1791-1793, 1996.

Cross-Reference

Neuroradiology: THE REQUISITES, pp 388-392, 424-431.

Comment

Giant cell reparative granulomas of the head and neck most commonly occur in the mandible and maxilla. Outside the jaw, the temporal bone and paranasal sinuses are the most common sites. It is a disease of adolescence, usually found in females. Mixed signal intensity and density (owing to blood products and hemosiderin), inhomogeneous enhancement, and lysis of the bone are typical. Most people believe the lesion to be due to traumatic or iatrogenic causes that incite intraosseous hemorrhage. The differential diagnosis often includes pigmented villonodular synovitis, giant cell tumors, ameloblastoma, aneurysmal bone cysts, fasciitis, and synovial chondromatosis.

The lesion is most often lytic with well- or ill-defined margins. It may be uni- or multilocular. On histology there are giant cells, fibroblastic cells, osteoid matrix, and foci of hemorrhage. The prognosis is excellent (as opposed to some of the other entities in the differential diagnosis).

Notes

Brucellosis

1. Tuberculous lymphadenitis, lymphoma, metastatic squamous cell carcinoma, infected branchial cleft cyst, and bacterial lymphadenitis.

2. *Brucella melitensis* (goats), *Brucella suis* (pigs), and *Brucella abortus* (cattle) are the main human pathogens. These are small gram-negative rods. Infection occurs through contact in the United States and through infected milk products in locations where pasteurization is not implemented.

3. Approximately 84%.

4. One hundred percent.

Reference

El-Desouki M: Skeletal brucellosis: assessment with bone scintigraphy, *Radiology* 181:415-418, 1991.

Cross-Reference

Neuroradiology: THE REQUISITES, p 405.

Comment

B. abortus is the most common type of brucellosis infection in North America. In endemic areas, musculoskeletal infection is the most common manifestation of disease, and the sacroiliac joints are affected most commonly—more so than the sternoclavicular joint and the costovertebral joints. This is a true zebra—one should have considered tuberculous adenitis in this case.

It is incredibly common in children to see adenopathy in the neck, often much greater than the usual 1-cm size criterion used for normality. Nodes as large as 2 cm may be seen in response to pharyngitis and ear infections, so the age of a patient with adenopathy (and his or her HIV status) should always be considered when reviewing a scan.

Notes

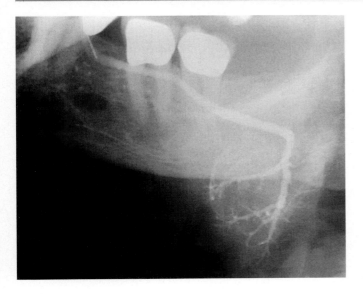

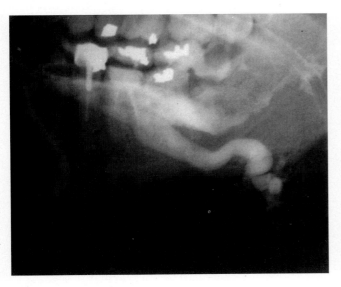
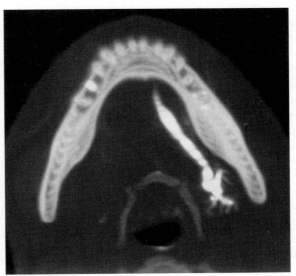

1. What are the imaging findings demonstrated in the figure in the upper left?

2. What causes ductal strictures?

3. If one saw punctate areas of contrast accumulation in the absence of the peripheral ductules, what would be the most likely diagnosis?

4. What are the indications for sialography?

Sialography and CT Sialography (Chronic Sialadenitis in Figure in Upper Left, Stricture in Figures in Lower Right and Lower Left)

1. Punctate areas of contrast enhancement around the peripheral ductules (which suggest peripheral ductal ectasia and cyst formation).

2. Sialolithiasis, chronic infection, and autoimmune sialadenitis.

3. Sjögren's syndrome or other autoimmune sialadenitis.

4. To demonstrate nonopaque calculi or causes of chronic sialadenitis when Sjögren's or Mikulicz's disease is not clinically apparent.

Reference

Szolar DH, Groell R, Braun H, Preidler K, Stiskal M, Kern R, Kainz J, Moelleken S, Stammberger H: Ultrafast computed tomography and three-dimensional image processing of CT sialography in patients with parotid masses poorly defined by magnetic resonance imaging, *Acta Otolaryngol* 116: 112-118, 1996.

Cross-Reference

Neuroradiology: THE REQUISITES, pp 417-418.

Comment

Sialography is a lot of fun and is still of some use to evaluate a patient who does not have calculi or masses in the salivary gland but has chronic salivary pain without a history of an autoimmune disorder. First you identify the ductal orifice by using lemon glycerin sticks and milking the gland forward. Then you cannulate the duct with dilators, praying fervently not to create a pseudotract in the mucosa that is not really the duct. Then you dilate the duct and stick your teeny-tiny catheter into the duct. You inject just enough Ethiodol (ethiodized oil) or Sinografin (diatrizoate meglumine; iodipamide meglumine) until the patient begins to feel discomfort. The patient bites down on the catheter, and you take your pictures and hope the contrast and the catheter stay in place. Postsialography CT produces beautiful scans of the ductal anatomy.

With ductal strictures or stones, patients experience discomfort and swelling in the gland, exacerbated by eating. Superimposed infection in the gland or duct is common. Sialodochoplasty can be performed for ductal strictures and can be combined with mechanical removal of the stone or laser extracorporeal shock wave lithotripsy to dissolve salivary stones. Alternatively, with anterior submandibular calculi, intraoral removal of the stones can be performed. With posterior calculi, removal of the gland may be performed with low morbidity.

Notes

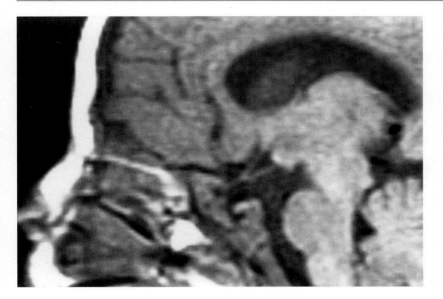
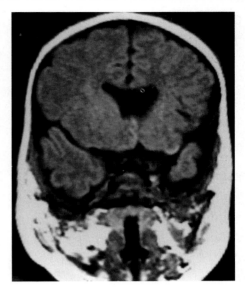
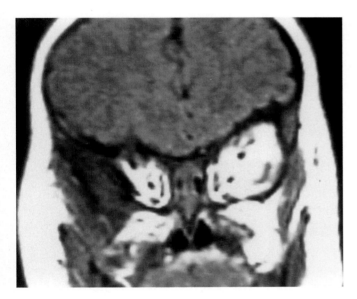

1. What are common causes of optic atrophy?

2. What intracranial congenital syndromes are associated with optic atrophy?

3. What is the common visual symptom associated with pituitary adenomas?

4. What congenital infection may cause optic atrophy?

Optic Atrophy Associated with Septooptic Dysplasia

1. Atherosclerosis, multiple sclerosis, sarcoidosis, vitamin deficiency, and neurodegenerative disorders.

2. Septooptic dysplasia (de Morsier's syndrome) and holoprosencephaly.

3. Bitemporal hemianopsia.

4. CMV, toxoplasmosis, or rubella infection.

Reference
Huber A: Genetic diseases of vision, *Curr Opin Neurol* 7:65-68, 1994.

Cross-Reference
Neuroradiology: THE REQUISITES, p 253.

Comment
Optic neuritis refers to an inflammatory condition of the nerves associated with decreased acuity with or without visual field defects. With chronic injury the optic disk appears pale and small on funduscopic evaluation, leading to a diagnosis of optic atrophy. Optic atrophy may be the sequela of metabolic disorders, toxins (lead, alcohol, mercury, arsenic), demyelinating processes (multiple sclerosis most commonly), infections (viruses usually), ischemia (older patients), vasculitides (temporal arteritis), vitamin deficiency (B_{12}, thiamine), histiocytosis, or congenital causes.

If you look histopathologically at patients with atherosclerosis of the central retinal artery, the most common findings are optic atrophy, atrophy of the retina, and cataracts. On Doppler ultrasound studies, no hemodynamic parameters or velocities are altered in patients with optic atrophy.

With the congenital causes, there are associations of optic atrophy with chromosome 3 anomalies (autosomal dominant optic atrophy), hereditary motor and sensory neuropathy type IV, linear nevus sebaceous syndrome, some mitochondrial myopathies, and Leber's hereditary optic neuropathy.

Notes

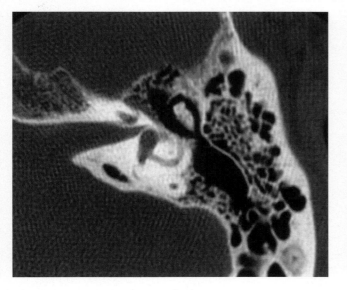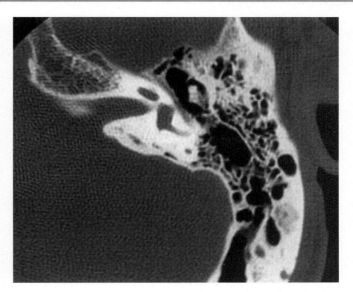

1. What are the pertinent findings?

2. When is malleus and incus fixation most commonly observed?

3. What is the most common mechanism for conductive hearing loss secondary to cholesteatomas?

4. What is the most common site of ossicular erosions?

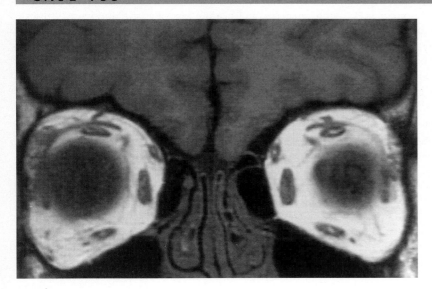

1. What normal structures are absent on this scan?

2. What are the congenital disorders associated with this finding?

3. What are the most common causes of loss of the sense of smell?

4. What is the classic tumor to affect the region of the ciliary nerves as they pass to the olfactory bulbs?

Malleus-Incus Fixation

1. Fusion of the joint between the malleus head and short process of the incus (figure on left) and lateral ligamentous ossification along the incus (figure on right).

2. With congenital (branchial cleft I) anomalies.

3. Ossicular erosions.

4. Distal incus, then stapes.

References
Gibb AG, Pang YT: Surgical treatment of tympanosclerosis, *Eur Arch Otorhinolaryngol* 252:1-10, 1995.

Swartz JD, Wolfson RJ, Marlowe FI, Popky GL: Postinflammatory ossicular fixation: CT analysis with surgical correlation, *Radiology* 154:697-700, 1985.

Cross-Reference
Neuroradiology: THE REQUISITES, pp 338-339.

Comment
Swartz and colleagues report that the vast majority of postinflammatory fixed ossicles are affected by fibrous tissue and/or hyalinization of cartilage, not by new bone formation. Suspensory ligaments and tendons may be involved and may be visualized as punctate or nodular calcification in the expected sites. The oval window may be closed by calcific debris indistinguishable from fenestral otosclerosis. This complication of otitis media may account for many of the noncholesteatomatous causes of a conductive hearing loss. Tympanosclerosis, of which postinflammatory ossicular fixation is an example, most commonly affects the tympanic membrane. Tympanosclerosis often exists in a setting of chronic otitis media and, along with atrophy of the pars tensa of the tympanic membrane, is a common sequela of middle ear infections and effusions. Trauma is another cause of tympanosclerosis. The lesion is rarely seen in the pars flaccida of the tympanic membrane and is usually found in the superior quadrants of the pars tensa. Ventilation tubes appear to predispose to tympanosclerosis. When the entity affects the middle ear ossicles, the malleus (situated apposed to the tympanic membrane) is most often affected. Stiffness of the tympanic membrane and malleus can cause an abnormal audiometric curve and a conductive hearing defect. The chronic inflammation of the middle ear is often bilateral.

Notes

Kallmann's Syndrome

1. The olfactory bulbs and tracts.

2. Kallmann's syndrome, holoprosencephaly, and septooptic dysplasia.

3. Viral upper respiratory tract infections and sinusitis.

4. Olfactory neuroblastoma/esthesioneuroblastoma.

Reference
Yousem DM, Geckle RJ, Bilker W, McKeown D, Doty RL: MR evaluation of patients with congenital hyposmia or anosmia, *AJR Am J Roentgenol* 166:439-444, 1996.

Cross-Reference
Neuroradiology: THE REQUISITES, pp 45-46.

Comment
Kallmann's syndrome consists of hypogonadotrophic hypogonadism associated with anosmia due to olfactory bulb aplasia. I was reproached in a letter to the editor in the *AJNR American Journal of Neuroradiology* for not giving first credit to the Maestre de San Juan, who described the entity 88 years before Kallmann in 1856. Sorry, but my Spanish is not very good, and I missed that reference. The syndrome is transmitted most frequently as an X-linked disorder characterized by infertility and anosmia. Reported cases of patients with cerebellar dysfunction, gait disturbances, spasticity, visual and extraocular motion abnormalities, and hearing loss suggest a multifaceted disease process. Kallmann's syndrome may be inherited as an autosomal dominant or recessive trait as well. It is 5 times more frequent in men than in women. Patients may or may not have development of olfactory sulci along their gyrus rectus region. Some believe that patients with Kallmann's syndrome have no olfactory neuroepithelium, whereas others believe that the olfactory axons simply fail to reach the prosencephalon and hence do not connect intracranially. The hypogonadism of Kallmann's syndrome is thought to be due to either a lack of cells that can express luteinizing hormone–releasing hormone (LHRH) or abnormal migration of the LHRH neurons from the olfactory placode in the nose to the hypothalamus.

When one looks at individuals with congenital anosmia, olfactory bulb and tract absence (68% to 84%) and hypoplasia (16% to 32%) are frequently seen. This patient had neither bulbs, tracts, nor "olfactory sulci."

Notes

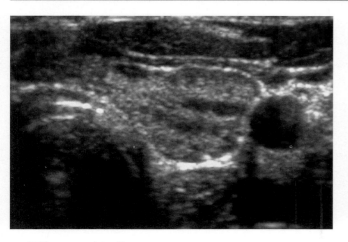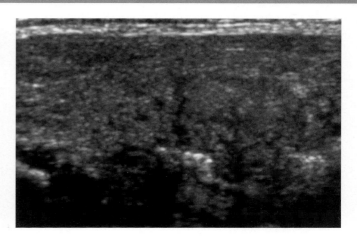

1. Who gets this disease?

2. Patients who have Hashimoto's thyroiditis are predisposed to what lesion of the thyroid gland?

3. What are the imaging features of Hashimoto's thyroiditis?

4. What is the etiology of Hashimoto's thyroiditis?

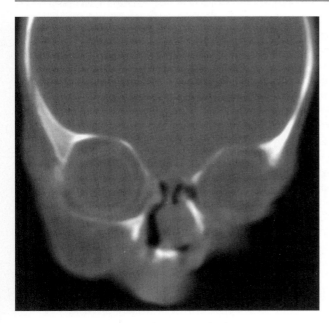

1. What is the grade of this nasal glioma?

2. What kind of attachment is present with the intracranial compartment?

3. Are nasal gliomas more commonly intranasal or extranasal?

4. Do nasal gliomas enhance?

Hashimoto's Thyroiditis

1. Middle-aged to elderly women most commonly. Frequently seen in the Japanese.

2. Primary thyroid lymphoma.

3. Nonspecific irregular architecture of the gland on ultrasound, CT, and MRI, with variable uptake (sometimes patchy) on nuclear medicine studies. The gland is often enlarged.

4. This is an autoimmune disorder in which the antigenic stimulus appears to be thyroglobulin or other thyroid cell antigens. It is associated with other autoimmune entities such as pernicious anemia, fibrosing mediastinitis, and sclerosing cholangitis.

Reference

Takashima S, Fukuda H, Tomiyama N, Fujita N, Iwatani Y, Nakamura H: Hashimoto thyroiditis: correlation of MR imaging signal intensity with histopathologic findings and thyroid function test results, *Radiology* 197:213-219, 1995.

Cross-Reference

Neuroradiology: THE REQUISITES, p 439.

Comment

Hashimoto's thyroiditis is an autoimmune disease in which circulating antithyroglobulin and microsomal antibodies are omnipresent. Follicular atrophy, fibrosis, enlargement of the gland, and firmness of the gland are seen. On MRI the T2W values of the gland with Hashimoto's thyroiditis are significantly higher than those of the glands of normal individuals. T1W values in lymphoma are greater than those in Hashimoto's thyroiditis. The study by Takashima and colleagues has suggested that as proton density (PD) and T2W signal intensity increase, TSH levels and follicular atrophy increase in untreated patients. Thus the higher the intensity, the greater the likelihood of hypothyroidism. Morphology may therefore reflect physiology. The authors also note that the higher the intensity on PD scans, the higher the rate of lymphoma.

A radioassay for thyroglobulin autoantibodies (TgAb) has been developed that can be used even on cytologic specimens. This may now be the most specific test for detecting Hashimoto's thyroiditis. Strangely enough, smoking may predispose a patient with Hashimoto's thyroiditis to the development of hypothyroidism. I say strangely enough because smoking seems to also affect patients with Graves' disease in the development of thyroid ophthalmopathy. Bottom line—don't smoke!

Notes

Nasal Glioma

1. Trick question—nasal gliomas are not tumors but are congenital rests.

2. Often (20%) there is a fibrous stalk to the meningeal surface, but effectively no communication is present.

3. Extranasal (60%). Thirty percent occur intranasally, and 10% are mixed.

4. Not usually.

Reference

Thomson HG, al-Qattan MM, Becker LE: Nasal glioma: is dermis involvement significant? *Ann Plast Surg* 34:168-172, 1995.

Cross-Reference

Neuroradiology: THE REQUISITES, pp 362-363.

Comment

Nasal gliomas are not neoplasms but should be thought of as congenital rests or heterotopic brain tissue with mature astrocytes. Some clinicians have adopted the term "nasal cerebral heterotopia," which seems more appropriate. Extranasal gliomas are diagnosed very early in life, but intranasal gliomas may be overlooked and not present until adulthood. Two theories have been espoused in the etiology of the nasal glioma: (1) Nasal gliomas occur due to entrapped neuroectodermal tissue left behind during calvarial closure, or (2) they represent cephaloceles that herniated downward but lost their blood supply and vital connection to the brain. Encephaloceles that maintain an open intracranial connection are much more common than nasal gliomas. Nasal gliomas are usually seen in the midline, and although they may be external to the nasal bones, there may be a fibrous connection to the nasal septum (hence a mixed extranasal and intranasal glioma). Strangely, high recurrence rates are reported.

Notes

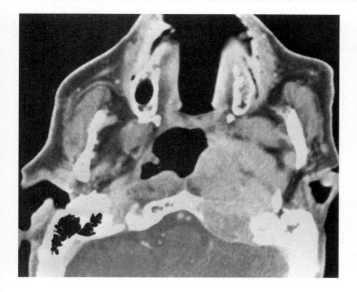
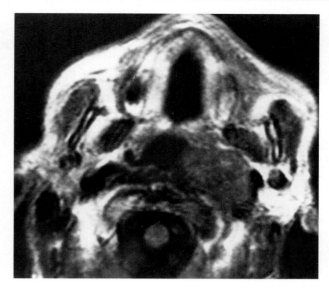
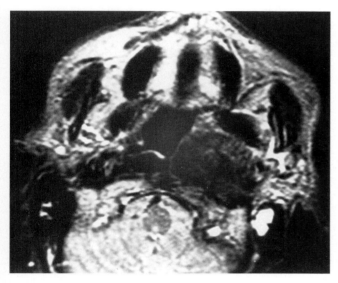

1. What are the signal intensity characteristics of amyloidomas on MRI?

2. What is the appearance on CT?

3. Where do they occur in the head and neck?

4. Where in the larynx do amyloidomas occur?

Amyloidoma*

1. Dark on T1W and T2W scans.

2. Dense with or without calcifications.

3. The larynx, followed by the oropharynx, trachea, orbit, nasopharynx, and oral cavity.

4. The supraglottic region submucosally.

Reference

Rodriguez-Romero R, Vargas-Serrano B, Cortina-Moreno B, Fernandez-Gallardo JM, Cervera-Rodilla JL: Calcified amyloidoma of the larynx, *AJNR Am J Neuroradiol* 17:1491-1494, 1996.

Cross-Reference

Neuroradiology: THE REQUISITES, p 398.

Comment

One can have localized amyloidomas without having systemic amyloidosis, although amyloidomas have been reported to occur in an isolated form in less than 15% of cases. When amyloidosis occurs in an organ-limited or focal form (without systemic manifestations), the most common sites are the head and neck, lung, heart, brain, and skin. The most common site of amyloid deposition in the head and neck is the larynx. Middle-aged men have a propensity for this disease. On imaging, the lesion has characteristic MRI findings (hypointense on all pulse sequences) and enhances minimally if at all—that would be unusual for most submucosal masses in the head and neck. Amyloidomas are usually hyperdense on unenhanced CT scans. Calcifications in a laryngeal mass should raise suspicions of chondrosarcomas, osteosarcomas, radiation effect, and tuberculosis—without enhancement, favor amyloid. Bone osteolysis with nonaggressive margins may be present.

Amyloidosis is yet another example of an immune system gone wrong, with immunoglobulins misdirected against the self and plasma cell proliferation. Congo red staining and green birefringence are the histologic hallmarks of amyloidosis.

Solitary head and neck extramedullary plasmacytomas occur in similar locations to amyloidomas (sinonasal cavity, nasopharynx, oropharynx, larynx, and oral cavity), usually in the submucosa. "Amyloid goiter" has also been reported in the thyroid gland. Treatment with radiation therapy is usually recommended.

Notes

---

* Figures for Case 186 courtesy Vijay Rao, MD.

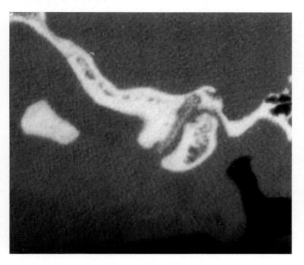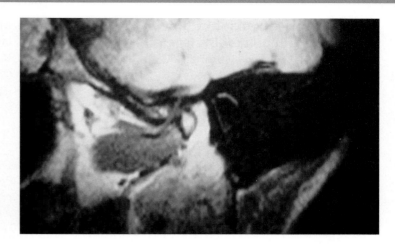

1. What is the usual management for painful syndromes associated with the temporomandibular joint?

2. What are the possible complications of Teflon-Proplast implants?

3. What surgical steps are taken before placement of a meniscal implant?

4. What are the commonest benign masses of the temporomandibular joint?

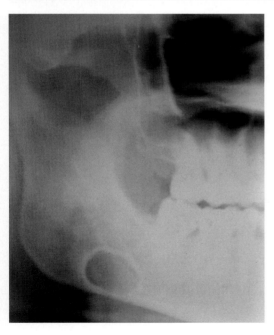

1. What causes a Stafne cyst?

2. Are Stafne cysts found in the maxilla?

3. What is their typical location with respect to the inferior alveolar canal?

4. What is the implication of a Stafne cyst?

Teflon-Proplast Implant of the Temporomandibular Joint (Migration)

1. Splinting and nonsteroidal antiinflammatory drugs, muscle relaxants, and soft diets.

2. Aseptic necrosis of the joint, migration of the implant, foreign body granuloma reaction, and arthrosis.

3. Disk plication to return it to its natural position, lysis of adhesions, and disk mobilization.

4. Osteochondromas and synovial chondromatosis.

Reference

Hansson LG, Eriksson L, Westesson P-L: Temporomandibular joint: MR evaluation after diskectomy, *Oral Surg Oral Med Oral Pathol Oral Radiol Endod* 74:801-810, 1992.

Cross-Reference

Neuroradiology: THE REQUISITES, pp 424-427.

Comment

The Teflon-Proplast meniscal replacement misadventure in the temporomandibular joint has cost the manufacturers a pretty penny. Several years after insertion of these implants the patients started to become symptomatic, in a fashion similar to some patients with breast implants. There began to be reports of granuloma formation, a foreign body autoimmune reaction to the implant, implant migration, implant fragmentation, and osteonecrosis of the condylar head.

On plain films expect to see single or multiple erosive changes in the mandibular condyle or temporal bone as one of the earliest features of foreign body giant cell reactions to the Teflon-Proplast implants. Sclerotic margins are variably present. Implant migration into the middle cranial fossa has been reported. (It's getting close here!)

Notes

Stafne Cyst of the Mandible*

1. A bone defect along the mandible's lingual surface presumed to be related to the submandibular gland because glandular tissue is within the cyst.

2. No.

3. Below the canal.

4. They are benign and do not necessitate treatment.

Reference

Gardner DG: An evaluation of reported cases of median mandibular cysts, *Oral Surg Oral Med Oral Pathol Oral Radiol Endod* 65:208-213, 1988.

Cross-Reference

Neuroradiology: THE REQUISITES, p 389.

Comment

The whole point here is not to go crazy sending in surgeons and bone doctors for what is a benign, normal variant—the impression on the mandible made by the submandibular gland. These cysts simulate unicameral bone cysts, Brown tumors, eosinophilic granulomas, and epidermoids. Other developmental cysts are much more common in the maxilla. The odontogenic cysts are obviously associated with the teeth (dentigerous cyst with an undescended tooth and radicular cyst with a carious tooth) but do not look at all like a Stafne cyst.

Notes

---

* Figure for Case 188 courtesy Mel (Muralidhar Mupparapu, DDS).

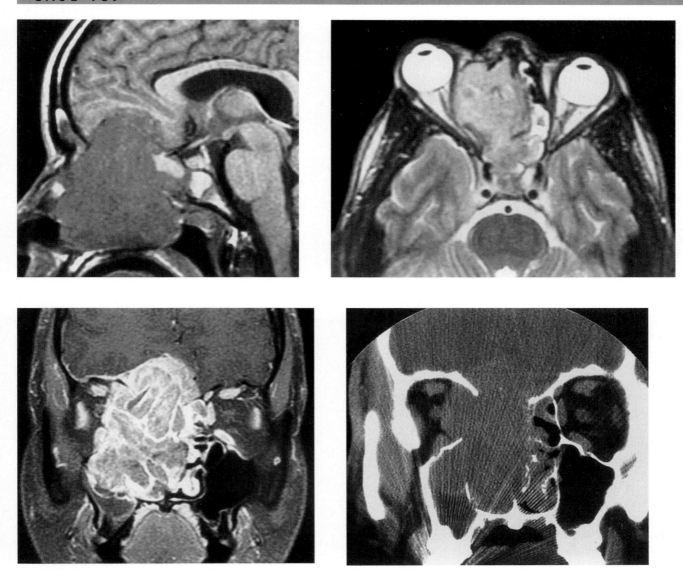

1. What does the differential diagnosis of this lesion, seen in a 20-year-old patient, include?

2. What single factor correlates best with prognosis in sinonasal sarcomas?

3. What is the median age for a rhabdomyosarcoma of the head and neck (half above and half below)?

4. Name the seven most common malignancies in children.

Rhabdomyosarcoma of the Sinonasal Cavity

1. Olfactory neuroblastoma, neuroendocrine tumor, lymphoma, and rhabdomyosarcoma.

2. Surgical margin.

3. Six years.

4. Leukemia, lymphoma, intracranial tumors, neuro-blastoma, Wilms' tumor, osteosarcoma, and rhabdomyosarcoma.

Reference

Min KW: Usefulness of electron microscopy in the diagnosis of "small" round cell tumors of the sinonasal region, *Ultrastruct Pathol* 19:347-363, 1995.

Cross-Reference

Neuroradiology: THE REQUISITES, pp 300-301.

Comment

Rhabdomyosarcomas are included in the dreaded "small round cell tumors" of the head and neck. These tumors include olfactory neuroblastomas, undifferentiated carcinomas, neuroendocrine tumors, melanomas, lymphomas, oat cell carcinoma, Ewing's sarcomas, and lymphoepitheliomas. If you get this diagnosis back on your cytologic specimen, forget about getting a final diagnosis without going to histology. Esthesioneuroblastomas and neuroendocrine tumors are particularly hard to differentiate, even with electron microscopy. Immunohistochemistry suggesting neuroblastic cells (dendritic processes, perikarya with granules) may be useful to the pathologists. The various small round cell tumors respond differently to chemotherapy and radiation, so a specific diagnosis may alter treatment.

Radiology can be helpful in that calcification might suggest an olfactory neuroblastoma, and MRI may help separate melanotic melanomas (high signal on T1W scans) from other lesions. Often lymphoma, neuroendocrine tumors, and rhabdomyosarcomas are indistinguishable on imaging. Rhabdomyosarcomas metastasize to the nodes in half of the patients and have hematogenous metastases in a similar percentage.

Note the orbital, dural, and intracranial involvement in this case.

Notes

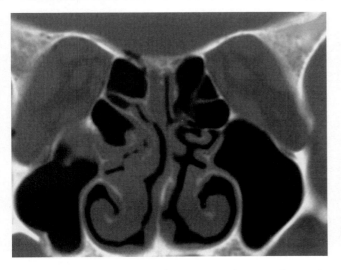
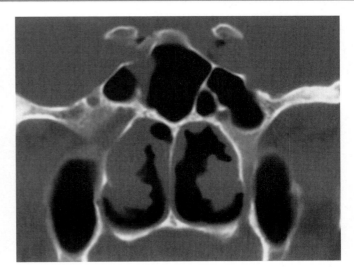

1. The fractures seen in this case predispose the patient to what?
2. What other bone is frequently fractured with the sphenoid sinus?
3. When one has a fracture of the posterior ethmoid or sphenoid sinus, what structures are at risk?
4. If this patient were to develop proptosis suddenly, what could be a source?

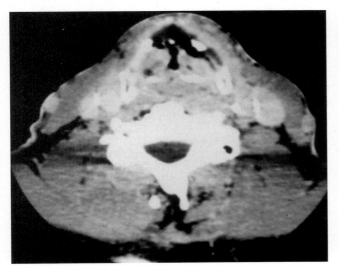
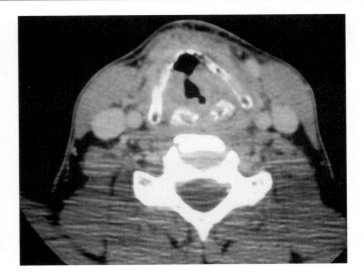

1. What are the common causes of cartilage collapse?
2. Is chondrified or ossified cartilage more vulnerable to chondronecrosis?
3. At what radiation dose does chondronecrosis become an issue?
4. What factors predispose to chondronecrosis from radiation therapy?

CASE 190

Fracture of the Cribriform Plate and Sphenoid Sinus

1. CSF leaks and meningitis.

2. The temporal bone.

3. The carotid artery, the optic nerve, and the cavernous sinus.

4. A carotid-cavernous fistula.

Reference
Dodson EE, Gross CW, Swerdloff JL, Gustafson LM: Transnasal endoscopic repair of cerebrospinal fluid rhinorrhea and skull base defects: a review of twenty-nine cases, *Otolaryngol Head Neck Surg* 111:600-605, 1994.

Cross-Reference
Neuroradiology: THE REQUISITES, pp 165-167.

Comment
Fractures of the skull base usually affect the more lateral structures than the paramedian ones. Nonetheless, one can fracture the sphenoid and basiocciput, though these are always in association with fractures that extend out laterally as well. The fractures are often bilateral and occur in the setting of severe head trauma, usually from a motor vehicle accident. The proximity of the optic nerves and carotid arteries to the basal skull bones can lead to serious neurovascular complications. In this case CSF leakage from the cribriform plate was a concern. Delayed CSF leakage and/or pneumocephalus can occur decades after the initial trauma to the patient. When it occurs, the patient may present with meningitis or rhinorrhea.

Notes

CASE 191

Chondronecrosis*

1. Trauma, iatrogenic (surgery) causes, and radiation.

2. Ossified cartilage.

3. At 6500 rad.

4. Exposed cartilage from surgery, poor vascularity to the tissue, and infection.

Reference
Moose BD, Greven KM: Definitive radiation management for carcinoma of the glottic larynx, *Otolaryngol Clin North Am* 30:131-143, 1997.

Cross-Reference
Neuroradiology: THE REQUISITES, pp 398-403, 408-410.

Comment
The variables that help predict successful radiation therapy include tumor bulk and the status of cord mobility. Impaired mobility denotes muscular or cricoarytenoid joint involvement and has a worse prognosis. Interruption of therapy for any reason leads to a worse outcome. Extensive cartilage invasion by the tumor or extension to the soft tissues of the neck is a contraindication to definitive radiotherapy because of the risk of inducing chondronecrosis.

Complications of radiotherapy should be in the 1% to 3% range for the treatment of T1-T2 glottic cancers. Acute reactions of laryngeal edema are to be expected, and dysphagia may occur. At higher dose fractionations, the rate of severe complications, including chondronecrosis, increases to up to 4%.

Radiation complications can be divided into two general types—acute and late. Acute complications are those that occur within the first 6 to 12 weeks of therapy and are due to radiation injury of rapidly dividing cells. These typically present with mucositis, edema, and sloughing. Late complications are due to small vessel vasculitis, fibrosis, and in severe cases necrosis. The tolerance of the laryngeal glottis, including the arytenoids, is 7000 rad in 200-rad fractions. Chondronecrosis is a risk even at that dose but usually does not occur until 3 to 12 months after therapy ends.

Fluorodeoxyglucose PET may be the most useful imaging study to differentiate chondronecrosis from recurrent or residual tumor. Chondronecrosis is treated with antibiotics, hyperbaric oxygen treatments, and steroids.

Notes

---

* Figures for Case 191 courtesy Hugh Curtin, MD.

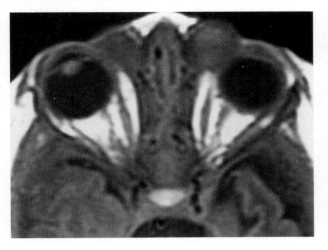 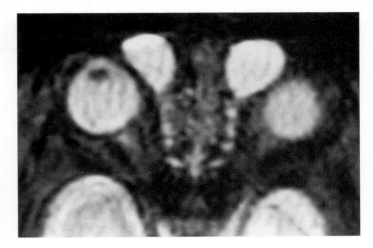

1. What are the typical CT findings of this entity?
2. How often does congenital obstruction of the lacrimal system occur?
3. What are the common histologies of lacrimal sac cancers?
4. Name three sphincters or valves within the lacrimal system.

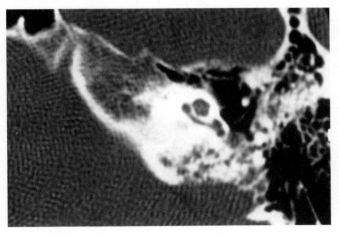 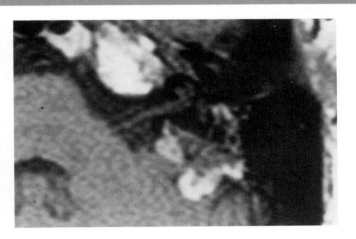

1. With what structure is this tumor associated?
2. Are the lesions sclerotic or lytic?
3. How do patients with this tumor present?
4. With what syndrome are endolymphatic sac tumors (ELSTs) associated?

Nasolacrimal Cystoceles

1. Cystic medial canthus mass, dilated nasolacrimal duct, and inferior nasal cavity mass.

2. Approximately 30% of the time.

3. Transitional cell and squamous cell carcinomas.

4. Valves of Bochdalek and Foltz lead to the lacrimal sac. Valves of Huschke and Rosenmüller are at the junction with the sinus of Maier and with the superomedial lacrimal sac. The valve of Krause (or Béraud) is at the inferior aspect of the sac. Within the nasolacrimal duct there are two valves—a superior valve of Taillefer and an inferior valve of Hasner that leads to the inferior meatus below the inferior turbinate.

Reference

Castillo M, Merten DF, Weissler MC: Bilateral nasolacrimal duct mucocele, a rare cause of respiratory distress: CT findings in two newborns, *AJNR Am J Neuroradiol* 14:1011-1013, 1993.

Cross-Reference

Neuroradiology: THE REQUISITES, p 361.

Comment

Neonatal obstructing lesions of the nasal cavity include hemangiomas, neurofibromas, cephaloceles, nasal gliomas, dermoids, and nasolacrimal duct cystoceles/mucoceles. Cystoceles/mucoceles usually develop due to congenital obstruction of the lower valves of Hasner of the nasolacrimal duct, but back-up can occur anywhere along the path of the developing nasolacrimal system. Therefore cysts can form at the punctum of the eye, within the lacrimal sac, in the upper lacrimal duct, or near the egress of tears at the inferior nasal turbinate.

Endonasal dacryocystoceles usually are seen under the inferior turbinate, causing a bulge in the medial canthal region. Neonates may have respiratory distress from the nasal airway compromise. Probing and marsupialization of the cyst may be required. On CT the nasolacrimal duct may be enlarged. The differential diagnosis clinically is dacryocystitis.

Notes

Papillary Endolymphatic Sac Tumor*

1. The endolymphatic sac/vestibular aqueduct.

2. Lytic, but they have bony matrix.

3. With hearing loss or tinnitus.

4. von Hippel–Lindau disease (approximately 7% of patients with von Hippel–Lindau disease develop ELSTs).

Reference

Mukherji SK, Albernaz VS, Lo WWM, Gaffey MJ, Megerian CA, Feghali JG, Brook A, Lewin JS, Lanzieri CF, Talbot JM, Meyer JR, Carmody RF, Weissman JL, Smirniotopoulos JG, Rao VM, Jinkins JR, Castillo M: Papillary endolymphatic sac tumors: CT, MR imaging, and angiographic findings in 20 patients, *Radiology* 202:801-808, 1997.

Cross-Reference

Neuroradiology: THE REQUISITES, pp 352-355.

Comment

This is a reasonably new entity that was formerly thought to be a metastasis to the temporal bone from an adenocarcinoma of unknown primary tumor, kidney, or thyroid origin. They are truly cystadenomatous tumors of the posterior petrous bone. These papillary lesions have been separated from the middle ear or mastoid "mixed" adenomas that are nondestructive and hypovascular. The papillary adenomatous tumors are hypervascular, have a spiculated or reticular appearance with calcified or bony matrix and rim, and aggressively infiltrate the posterior temporal bone. The lesion does not metastasize. Dural invasion may occur early in the tumor's course. Blood products in cysts or intratumoral hemorrhage collects, and this, coupled with the bony matrix, may lead to variable signal intensity patterns on MRI. High signal on T1W scans is seen in 80% of cases, and enhancement is the rule. The left side is more commonly involved than the right, and patients often present with facial nerve palsies and tinnitus. Flow voids may be seen within the lesion on MRI and correspond to large external carotid artery branches (ascending pharyngeal and stylomastoid artery tributaries). The differential diagnosis of such aggressive posterior temporal bone lesions would include metastases, cholesterol granulomas, paragangliomas, hemangiopericytomas, and chondroid lesions. When the imaging findings are coupled with the characteristic location centered at the endolymphatic sac, a papillary adenomatous tumor becomes the best diagnosis. Bilateral ELSTs should raise the possibility of von Hippel–Lindau disease.

Notes

---

* Figures for Case 193 courtesy William W.N. Lo, MD.

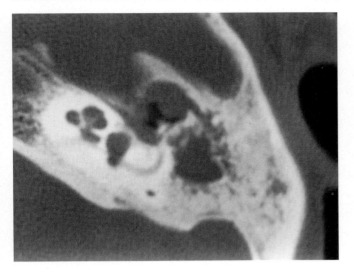 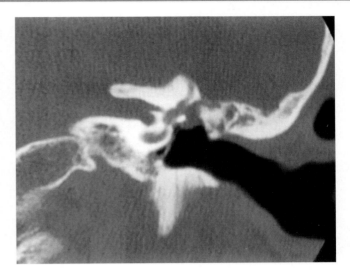

1. In this patient with chronically draining ear, what is the best diagnosis?

2. What are the potential complications of acquired cholesteatomas?

3. Which semicircular canal is most commonly affected by cholesteatomas?

4. What are the imaging features of acquired cholesteatomas on MRI?

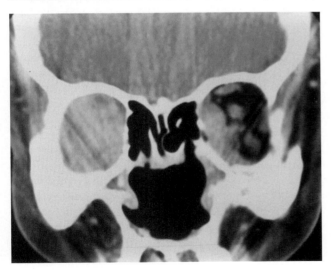

1. What are the manifestations of this entity in the head and neck (non-CNS)?

2. How often are the brain and/or meninges involved?

3. What triad defines Wegener's granulomatosis?

4. What are the manifestations of Wegener's granulomatosis in the brain?

Labyrinthine Fistula with Facial Nerve Dehiscence from a Cholesteatoma

1. Acquired cholesteatoma.

2. Labyrinthine fistulas, facial nerve fistulas, invasion of the tegmen tympani with intracranial extent, ossicular erosion, vascular invasion, and automastoidectomy.

3. The lateral semicircular canal.

4. Intermediate signal intensity on T1W scans and intermediate signal intensity on T2W scans with peripheral contrast enhancement. Most cholesteatomas do not significantly enhance.

Reference

Mafee MF: MRI and CT in the evaluation of acquired and congenital cholesteatomas of the temporal bone, *J Otolaryngol* 22:239-248, 1993.

Cross-Reference

Neuroradiology: THE REQUISITES, pp 342-344.

Comment

The evaluation of an acquired cholesteatoma does not stop when you have identified scutum erosion and have therefore suggested a cholesteatoma. In fact, CT is relatively inaccurate for distinguishing acute or chronic otitis media and granulation tissue from acquired cholesteatomas—clinicians rely on otoscopy. What they really want is knowledge of the integrity of the labyrinth, facial nerve canal, semicircular canal, tegmen tympani, sigmoid sinus plate, and carotid wall. They are trying to avoid a surgical disaster. They also want to make sure that there is not an underlying vascular mass. CT is better for evaluating the integrity of the semicircular canals (97% accuracy, 100% sensitivity) than it is for evaluating the facial nerve canal (75% accuracy due to high false negative rates, 66% sensitivity). In normal ears the rate of facial canal dehiscence approaches 50% by microscopy.

Notes

Wegener's Granulomatosis

1. Sinusitis, orbital granulomas, epistaxis, glottic or subglottic stenosis, optic neuropathy, nasal septal erosion, conjunctivitis, scleritis, uveitis, and mastoiditis. Ocular disease is seen in 40%.

2. Less than 5% of the time.

3. Respiratory tract necrotizing granulomas, vasculitis, and glomerulonephritis.

4. Vasculitis with infarcts, dural enhancement, brainstem and white matter foci of increased intensity on T2W scans, hemorrhage, cerebritis, and superimposed infections.

Reference

Provenzale JM, Allen NB: Wegener granulomatosis: CT and MR findings, *AJNR Am J Neuroradiol* 17:785-792, 1996.

Cross-Reference

Neuroradiology: THE REQUISITES, pp 297, 317.

Comment

Wegener's granulomatosis is a systemic disease with protean manifestations in the head and neck and brain. The disease appears to be immune related, with autoantibodies directed against proteinases of neutrophils and monocytes suggestive of active disease. Midline lethal granuloma (malignant midline reticulosis) is the classic differential diagnosis in the sinonasal cavity—both entities affect the nasal septum early on, leading to a "saddle nose deformity" as a result of erosion and collapse. Midline lethal granuloma often progresses to lymphoma and has recently been reclassified as a premalignant lesion. Wegener's granulomatosis is often not very bright on T2W MRI, making it unusual for an inflammatory condition. Wegener's granulomatosis can affect the pituitary stalk and cause diabetes insipidus.

Pyoderma gangrenosum (a skin lesion associated with Wegener's granulomatosis), vasculitis causing strokes, laryngotracheal stenosis, rhinitis, nasal obstruction, and mucosal ulceration may lead to head and neck imaging in a patient with Wegener's granulomatosis. Cyclophosphamide and steroids result in high control rates for this disease.

Notes

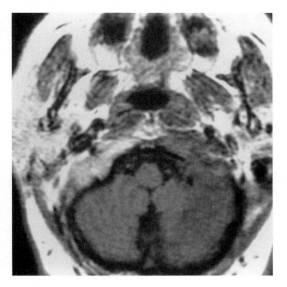

1. Where is the abnormality located?
2. What is the most common lesion here? Describe its mechanism.
3. What symptoms are elicited from patients with this lesion?
4. What are the most common tumors to metastasize to the occipital condyle?

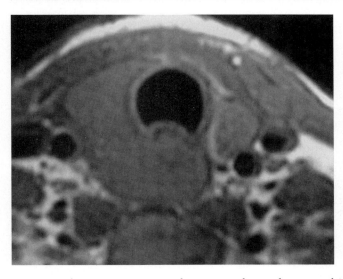 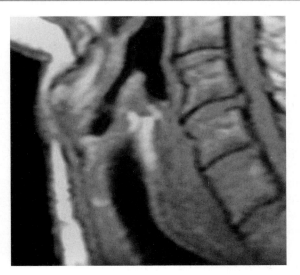

1. Does this tumor seem to be mucosal or submucosal in origin?
2. What are the most common histologies of mucosal cancers of the upper esophagus?
3. What is the most likely submucosal mass of the esophagus?
4. Where do granular cell tumors (myoblastomas) occur in the head and neck?

Metastasis to the Left Occipital Condyle

1. In the left occipital condyle.

2. Fracture. Type I—axial loading injury in association with ipsilateral flexion; type II—basilar skull fracture extending into the condyle from a blow to the skull; and type III—avulsion fracture from a combination of contralateral head flexion and rotation.

3. Occipital headaches, neck pain, tongue fasciculations, and weakness.

4. Those in gastrointestinal sites, followed by those in the prostate.

Reference
Loevner LA, Yousem DM: The overlooked occipital condyle: a missed case treasure trove, *Radiographics* 17:1111-1121, 1997.

Cross-Reference
Neuroradiology: THE REQUISITES, pp 436-437.

Comment
The craniovertebral junction and the occipital condyles are usually included in all brain and cervical spine radiologic studies, but because they are at the edges of the films they are frequently overlooked. This leads to a high rate of underreported occipital condyle lesions. The proximity to the hypoglossal canal, located at the anterior margin of the occipital condyles (transmitting the twelfth cranial nerve), and the jugular foramen, located antero-lateral and superior to the occipital condyles (transmitting cranial nerves nine through eleven), accounts for the proclivity toward lower cranial neuropathies associated with condylar lesions. Fractures are also commonly overlooked here—coronal CT reconstructions and careful review of axial scans help to avoid missing this diagnosis. For neoplasms, carefully review sagittal and axial T1W scans for normal bright marrow fat in the condyles.

In this case the patient shows abnormal tissue in the prevertebral tissue on the left side and growing into the inferior jugular foramen. Keen eyes will detect abnormal signal in the left cerebellum. This bone metastasis grew through the dura and into the brain.

Notes

Granular Cell Tumor of the Upper Esophagus

1. Submucosal, owing to its eccentric location.

2. Squamous cell carcinoma and adenocarcinoma. (Recall Barrett's esophagus.)

3. Leiomyoma, followed by lipoma.

4. In the tongue, skin, and subcutaneous tissues.

Reference
Boncoeur-Martel M-P, Loevner LA, Yousem DM, Elder DE, Weinstein GS: Granular cell tumor ("myoblastoma") of the cervical esophagus: findings on MR, *AJNR Am J Neuroradiol* 17:1794-1797, 1996.

Cross-Reference
Neuroradiology: THE REQUISITES, p 401.

Comment
This case is unusual because the gastrointestinal tract is an unusual place for granular cell tumors, the esophagus is an unusual place in the gastrointestinal tract for this lesion, and the proximal portion of the esophagus is not as commonly affected as the distal portion of the esophagus. Call it a purple-spotted zebra, I guess. The tumor is of neuroectodermal derivation and affects women more than men, blacks more than whites. Granular cell tumors are benign, and wide local excision (because they may be stuck to adjacent muscular tissue) is usually sufficient treatment. They usually occur in young adults along the lateral aspect or tip of the oral tongue, although floor of mouth granular cell myoblastomas are also reported.

Notes

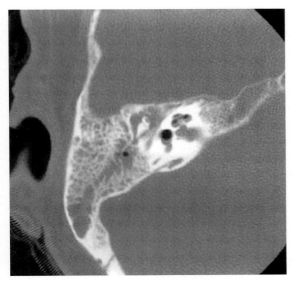

1. Where is there abnormal air in this case?

2. For what should one search upon seeing air there?

3. What is implied by the presence of air in the vestibule postoperatively?

4. What is the cause of this patient's pneumolabyrinthitis?

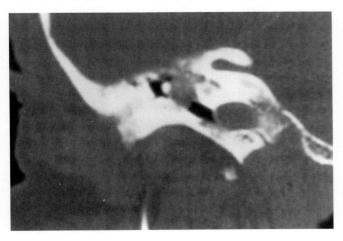 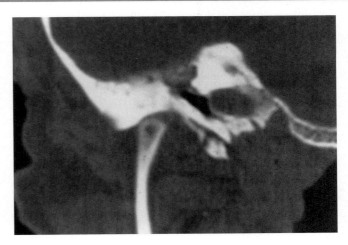

1. If this were seen in the vertebral body, what would be the most likely diagnosis?

2. What nerve emanates from the geniculate ganglion?

3. At the geniculate ganglion, what are the most common tumors?

4. What is an intratemporal benign vascular tumor?

Ossicular Erosions and Pneumolabyrinthitis from Chronic Otitis Media

1. In the vestibule and cochlea.

2. A fracture because trauma—or an air leak of some type—is one of the most common causes.

3. A perilymphatic fistula from middle ear to inner ear.

4. It is probably inflammatory because there is an erosion in the malleus head and no evidence of surgery or trauma.

Reference

Lyos AT, Marsh MA, Jenkins HA, Coker NJ: Progressive hearing loss after transverse temporal bone fracture, *Arch Otolaryngol Head Neck Surg* 121:795-799, 1995.

Cross-Reference

Neuroradiology: THE REQUISITES, pp 342-343.

Comment

Trauma is the most common cause of pneumolabyrinth. However, this patient had no history of trauma and instead had an infection with gas-producing organisms. Trauma, surgery, and congenital dehiscences can predispose one to developing air in the bony labyrinth. Transverse fractures of the temporal bone appear to have the highest rate of pneumolabyrinth. Usually air in the labyrinth implies a communication with the middle ear cavity and therefore a perilymphatic fistula. Hearing loss is usually pretty profound with a perilymphatic fistula. Often the site of opening between inner and middle ear is the round or oval window. This must be repaired quickly to avoid chronic ear problems, permanent hearing loss, vestibular symptoms, and/or meningitis. With middle ear disease the spread to the inner ear is most commonly through the oval or round windows; however, fistula to the semicircular canal is another option. Causes may be bacterial or viral.

Notes

Geniculate Ganglion Hemangioma

1. A hemangioma.

2. The greater superficial petrosal nerve.

3. Schwannoma and hemangioma, followed by epidermoids.

4. A term used to capture cavernous hemangiomas, capillary hemangiomas, and vascular malformations of the temporal bone. They typically occur along the course of the facial nerve.

Reference

Lo WWM, Shelton C, Waluch V, Solti-Bohman LG, Carberry JN, Brackmann DE, Wade CT: Intratemporal vascular tumors: detection with CT and MR imaging, *Radiology* 171:445-448, 1989.

Cross-Reference

Neuroradiology: THE REQUISITES, pp 339-340, 347-348.

Comment

When intratemporal vascular tumors produce intratumoral bony spicules, they are called ossifying hemangiomas. The tumors favor the geniculate ganglion region yet may occur anywhere along the facial nerve. Patients most frequently present with a Bell's palsy, but occasionally the presenting symptoms suggest an eighth nerve lesion—tinnitus and/or hearing loss. They cause symptoms at a smaller size than do schwannomas.

Notes

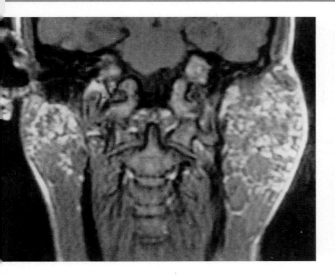
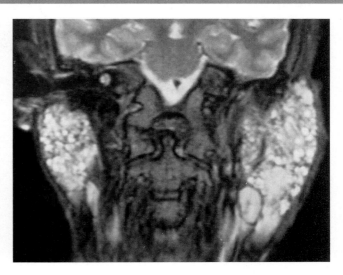
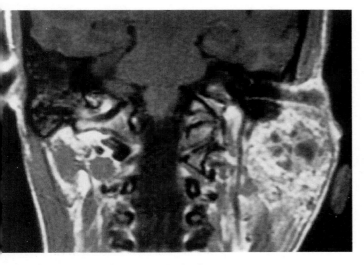

1. Define sialectasia and sialodochitis.

2. To what are patients with Sjögren's syndrome predisposed?

3. What is Schirmer's test?

4. Which duct is easier to cannulate, Stensen's duct or Wharton's duct?

5. Can I get the last (801st) question in this book correct?

Sjögren's Parotitis

1. Dilated ducts and inflamed ducts.

2. Lymphoma. The rate is three times that of control subjects and the tumor may be extraparotid or intraparotid.

3. A paper test of lacrimation to determine tear production. It is decreased in Sjögren's syndrome.

4. Stensen's (parotid).

5. Yes

Reference

Izumi M, Eguchi K, Ohki M, Uetani M, Hayashi K, Kita M, Nagataki S, Makamura T: MR imaging of the parotid gland in Sjögren's syndrome: a proposal for new diagnostic criteria, *AJR Am J Roentgenol* 166:1483-1487, 1996.

Cross-Reference

Neuroradiology: THE REQUISITES, pp 300, 418.

Comment

Sjögren's syndrome (xerostomia, keratoconjunctivitis sicca, and collagen vascular disease) is a disease of middle-aged women. Heterogeneous signal intensity on MRI of the parotid gland with or without cysts and nodules is the norm with this disease. The causes of sialectasia include stone disease, chronic sialadenitis, sarcoidosis, and ductal obstructive lesions.

Sjögren's syndrome and lupus erythematosus can coexist, and both can cause a vasculitis that can affect the brain or optic nerves. The diagnosis is usually made by the demonstration of antinuclear antibodies SS-A or SS-B in the blood, seen with both conditions in most cases. A labial biopsy may also be performed to confirm the clinical diagnosis of Sjögren's syndrome—lymphocytes that are T cell, CD4 positive are usually seen.

Although the concentration of albumin, IgA, cystatins, and other proteins is increased in the saliva of patients with Sjögren's syndrome, the output of total saliva is decreased. Therefore the total defense system of the saliva is decreased in the mouth, accounting for the problems of poor dental hygiene in patients with the syndrome.

A fascinating clinical tidbit: Frey's syndrome (auriculotemporal syndrome) involves sweating and flushing of the skin when the patient salivates. It is due to an injury of a branch of the third division of the fifth cranial nerve (the auriculotemporal nerve), usually seen after parotidectomy.

Ta-dah!

Notes